AIDS and Beyond

Dietary and Lifestyle Guidelines for New Viral and Bacterial Diseases

By Michio Kushi with Alex Jack
Foreword by Edward Esko

One Peaceful World Press
Becket, Massachusetts

Note to the Reader:

It is advisable for the reader to seek the guaidance of a physician or other appropriate health care professional before implementing the approach to health suggested in this book. It is essential that any reader who has any reason to suspect serious illness contact a physician promptly. Neither this nor any other book should be used as a substitute for professional medical care or treatment.

AIDS and Beyond
© 1995 by Michio Kushi and Alex Jack

For further information on mail-order sales, wholesale or retail discounts, distribution, translations, and foreign rights, please contact the publisher:

One Peaceful World Press
P.O. Box 10
Leland Road
Becket, MA 01223
U.S.A.

Telephone (413) 623-2322
Fax (413) 623-8827

First Edition: January 1995
10 9 8 7 6 5 4 3 2 1

ISBN 1–882984–09–9
Printed in U.S.A.

Contents

New Viral and Bacterial Diseases

Emerging Viral Diseases

Disease	Region/Outbreak	Transmission	Dietary Factor	Social Factor
AIDS	USA, 1981-, Africa, global, 1990s	Sexual contact, transfusions	Sugar, tropical foods, oil, dairy, fat	Ecological imbalance, antibiotic use
Argentine hemorrhagic fever	Argentina, 1958-	Rodents	Meat, sugar	Modern farming
Dengue	Cuba, 1981, Asia, Africa, Australia	Mosquitoes, monkey/human	Sugar, fruit, dairy	Urbanization, open water
Ebola hemorrhagic fever	Zaire, Sudan, 1976-	Unknown	Sugar, dairy, oil, fat	Ecological imbalance
Hantaan	Asia, U.S., 1993-	Rodents	Meat, sugar	Monoculture
Hepatitis C & E	Tropics, 1990s	Waterborne	Meat, sugar	Transfusions
Human T Cell Leukemia	Caribbean, 1979, Japan 1983, global	Humans	Sugar, fruit, dairy, oil, fat	Medical tech/ transfusions
Influenza (H-3 and New H-1)	Global, 1968-, 1977-	Fowl, swine, humans	Meat, sugar, dairy, oil, fat	Duck-pig agriculture
Lassa fever	West Africa, 1969-	Rodents	Sugar, dairy	Mining
Marburg disease	Germany, 1967, Africa, 1975	Monkeys	Sugar, dairy, fruit, oil, fat	Polio vaccine, hospitals
Rift Valley fever	Egypt, 1977	Camels, cattle, mosquitoes	Sugar, dairy, fruit, oil, fat	Dams, irrigation
Yellow fever	Nigeria, 1986, Kenya, 1992	Monkeys, mosquitoes	Fruit, sugar, chocolate, dairy	Modern farming, medical technology

Emerging Bacterial Diseases

Disease	Region/Outbreak	Transmission	Dietary Factor	Social Factor
Cholera	Tropics, 1980s-90s	Waterborne	Sugar, dairy	Antibiotics
E. Coli infections	U.S., Mexico, S.E. Asia, 1980s-	Food-, air-, waterborne	Sugar, dairy, fat, oil, fruit	Undercooked meat/poultry
Gonorrhea	Philippines, 1975, global, 1980s-90s	Sexual contact	Meat, sugar, dairy, oil, fat	Antibiotic resistance
?Gulf War syndrome	U.S., 1991-	War-, hospital-borne	Meat, sugar, dairy, oil, fat	Nerve agents, vaccines
Legionnaire's disease	U.S., 1976-	Air- and water-borne	Meat, sugar, dairy, oil, fat	Airconditioning, ducts
Lyme disease	U.S., Europe, Australia, 1980s-90s	Deer tick	Sugar, chocolate, fruit, fat	Urbanization, pesticides
Pneumonia	U.K., U.S., 1963, global, 1980s-90s	Airborne	Meat, sugar, dairy, oil, fat	Resistance to antibiotics
Salmonella	Iran, 1963-73, global, 1980s-90s	Food-, air-borne	Meat, sugar, dairy, oil, fat	Contaminated meat/poultry
Shigella dysentery	Japan, 1955, Tropics, 1980s-90s	Water-, air-, food-borne	Sugar, milk, tropical foods	Resistance to antibiotics
Staph infections	Global, 1980s-90s	Airborne	Sugar, fruit	Antibiotics
Strep A infections (necrotizing fasciitis)	Australia, 1960s, U.K., U.S., 1994	Air-, hospital-borne	Sugar, chocolate, dairy, fruit, oil, fat	Resistance to antibiotics
Tuberculosis	Global, 1980s-1990s	Air-, hospital-borne	Fruit, sugar, dairy, fat, oil	Antibiotic resistance, AIDS

Source: *AIDS and Beyond* by Michio Kushi and Alex Jack, © 1995

Foreword

Fifteen years ago, the East West Foundation presented the third of its annual cancer conferences in Boston. The speakers included Michio Kushi and other macrobiotic educators, along with a distinguished panel of doctors and researchers, including Drs. Anthony Sattilaro and Robert Mendelsohn. I also had the privilege of speaking, and in my remarks, pointed to the decline of infectious disease and the subsequent rise of lifestyle-caused illnesses during the 20th century.

The consensus was essentially that since the plagues of the 20th century—cancer and heart disease—were a product of personal dietary and lifestyle choices, modern medicine could offer little in the way of a *fundamental* solution. The antibiotics and other treatments developed in response to infectious diseases were of little or no use against these modern lifestyle-induced conditions and, therefore, what was needed was a new medicine that incorporated an understanding of lifestyle and diet.

However, with the appearance of AIDS several years later, it soon became clear that the problem of infectious disease was far from over. By the early '80s, Michio Kushi and other macrobiotic teachers were frequently being invited to address AIDS conferences in New York City and other parts of the country. Hundreds of persons with AIDS had adopted a macrobiotic lifestyle and experienced noticeable improvements in the quality of their lives.

At a symposium entitled, "Meeting the Challenge of AIDS: Professional and Community Response," held in the autumn of 1983 at Hunter College in New York, Mr. Kushi delivered the following message to an audience that included many persons with AIDS:

> I wish to tell all AIDS friends that there is a way to recover from their present suffering, unless the disorder if too far advanced. The way to recover is actually quite simple, once proper understanding has been established. Many AIDS friends are frightened with uncertainty about the future. Many people in society are also anxious and afraid of possible contact and spread of AIDS among their friends, family, and community. However, it is, in another sense, a golden opportunity for inner reflection by everyone . . . . Through this critical experience, I trust everyone will develop a vision of the future which is one peaceful world through maximum health and highest spirit.

As you will discover in the pages of *AIDS and Beyond*, infectious diseases may be to the 21st century what cancer and heart disease were to the 20th century. Yet, there are some rays of hope. The vanguard of modern research is now pointing in a holistic macrobiotic direction. The failure of modern virus theory to fully explain or account for AIDS is leading to the self-reflection that Mr. Kushi called for at the beginning of the AIDS crisis. Not only are individual dietary, environmental, and lifestyle factors being suspected as primary in the development of AIDS, as well as in the appearance of new viral and bacterial infections, but civilization's continuing disruption of the planet itself is now being viewed as a possible cause of these present and future epidemics.

AIDS and Beyond brings these facts to light, and in so doing focuses public attention on the critical importance of planetary ecology in human health and well-being, as well as the all-important role of diet and lifestyle in strengthening natural immunity. It also presents the basic dietary and lifestyle guidelines so urgently needed to reverse this crisis and avert planet-wide catastrophe.

Edward Esko
Becket, Massachusetts

Introduction
The Evolutionary Crisis

Humanity faces an evolutionary crisis. The continued destruction of the earth's natural environment, the possible onset of global warming, the spread of political and economic instability, and the emergence of AIDS and other viral and bacterial epidemics imperil the continued existence of our species, as well as many others. All around us we see millions of people in apparent good health, and we assume that *homo sapiens* will survive and multiply in the 21st century. However, just as the Soviet Union—mighty and seemingly indestructible just a few years ago—collapsed, humanity as a whole may collapse as personal, social, and planetary health systems are stretched beyond their limits.

In fact, the magnitude of the crisis has led some people to conclude that the earth itself is terminally ill. Metaphors comparing some of these global problems to cancer, heart disease, and AIDS are commonplace. The buildup of toxic deposits in the land is likened to the development of tumors in vital organs. The pollution of streams and rivers shares a resemblance to leukemia and lymphoma. The thinning of the ozone layer, leading to the weakening of many plants and animals, is like loss of the planet's natural immunity.

Clearly, humanity and the planet as a whole are in urgent need of healing. For many years, the macrobiotic community has been saying that the outer environment reflects the inner environment and that the key to our dilemma is a return to a more natural way of life, including a more natural way of eating. Personal health cannot be separated from planetary health, and wholesome natural foods are the bridge between the two.

During the last twenty years, dietary awareness has increased throughout modern society. The scientific and medical professions have discovered the connection between the modern way of eating and heart disease and cancer—the two leading causes of death—and issued dietary guidelines moving in a healthier direction. Largely as a result of changing toward a low-fat, high-fiber diet, the death rate from cardiovacular disease has dropped 40 percent in the United States. Cancer rates as a whole are still climbing; however, some individual malignancies are beginning to peak. We can expect further drop offs in selected cancers in the next decade as recent dietary changes take effect.

Despite the success in reducing chronic diseases, infectious diseases are on the rise and threaten to become the new plagues of the 21st century. Since the early 1980s, AIDS has encircled the globe, moving from the homosexual into the heterosexual population and affecting millions of people. About 22 million people are presently infected, and the World Health Organization expects up to 40 million to be infected by the year 2000. In sub-Saharan Africa, 94 percent of AIDS cases are the result of sexual intercourse between men and women, and in the United States, the rate of heterosexual transmission jumped 130 percent last year. In tropical regions of Africa, South Asia, and Southeast Asia, the total number of cases has reached 10-30 percent in some regions, already posing catastrophic social and medical problems and threatening these societies with collapse. In the United States, AIDS has increased 77 percent among adolescents in the last two years, and around the world the childhood mortality rate from AIDS is projected to triple by 2010.

The failure of the conventional approach to treating AIDS has become apparent. Despite billions of dollars of research and the time and energy of thousands of scientists, no effective vaccine has been developed. AZT and other drugs have proved to be worthless, or even counterproductive.

8

Meanwhile, within the scientific community, the whole medical strategy of dealing with AIDS has come under review. Increasingly, researchers are questioning the theory that a single virus is the primary cause of AIDS and that vaccines and drugs are the best way to combat it. Signs of a change in orientation include the following:

• By the end of 1992, over 100 cases of AIDS had been documented in which the patients were free of HIV, the Human Immunodeficiency Virus associated with the disease.

• Dr. Luc Montagnier, discoverer of HIV and professor and director of virology at the Pasteur Institute in Paris, France, announced that he believed HIV was no longer sufficient to cause AIDS. "I think we should put the same weight on co-factors as we have on HIV," he told the Eighth International Conference on AIDS in 1992. He identified a new strain of *Mycoplasma*, a bacterium, as a likely co-factor and speculated that a virulent form of this organism developed from the overuse of antibiotics, especially tetracycline.

• Dr. Robert Gallo, the co-discoverer of HIV and chief of the Laboratory of Tumor Cell Biology at the National Institutes of Health, also questioned whether HIV is the sole cause of AIDS. "I also intuitively agree with the idea that co-factors for HIV progression itself also exist," he wrote in his book *Virus Hunting*. He identified HTLV-1, the Human T-Cell Leukemia Virus, as a probable co-factor and stated there may be others, as well as a variety of social and environmental conditions that modified susceptibility to infection.

• In 1993, a Group for the Scientific Reappraisal of the HIV/AIDS Hypothesis, comprised of several hundred scientists including many AIDS researchers, issued an international appeal calling for a thorough reappraisal of the viral hypothesis. They hypothesized that AIDS was caused by preexisting immunosuppressive factors including drug use, overmedicalization, and improper diet.

• In 1994 Dr. Bernard Fields, the chairman of the department of microbiology and molecular genetics at Harvard Medical School, presented a blueprint in the scientific journal *Nature* calling for a fundamental redirection in the government's approach to AIDS. Questioning the model of developing vaccines and drugs, Dr. Fields called for efforts toward learning the basics of the disease.

• At the tenth International Conference on AIDS in Yokohama, Japan, in August, 1994, the coordinator of AIDS research in the United States announced a shift toward basic research in the immune response, as opposed to focusing on the virus, and a cut in spending on clinical trials of potential drugs.

From the beginning of the AIDS epidemic, we have been saying within the macrobiotic community that modern dietary, lifestyle, and environmental factors are the primary cause of the disease. A harmful virus, and possibly other virulent microorganisms, are associated with the majority of cases. However, susceptibility to infection in any given instance depends upon our natural immunity. This, in turn, depends on many factors, the most important of which is daily way of eating. While there is little study on preventing AIDS with diet, research has shown that diet may be helpful in prolonging life. In the 1980s, researchers at Boston University studied men with AIDS who adopted a macrobiotic diet and found that their quality of life improved and their average survival rate exceeded that of all other groups under review.

In the next several years, modern science and medicine very likely will discover diet as a primary cause of immune-deficiency just as it discovered diet as the underlying cause of heart disease and cancer. In this book, we present a comprehensive approach to AIDS and other viral and bacterial diseases based on the macrobiotic understanding of health and upon current scientific and medical research. The emphasis is on *prevention* of AIDS through changes in diet and lifestyle that increase our natural immunity to disease and infection. However, in the last chapter, we present guidelines for *recovery* for those who already have AIDS or who have tested positive for HIV. Depending on the individual case, these guidelines may be helpful in reversing the course of the disease, in prolonging life expectancy, or in improving the quality of life.

The rapid spread of AIDS around the world is alarming.

However, it is becoming clear that AIDS is just the beginning of a new cycle of epidemics. In the last several years, a wave of infectious diseases has emerged and is now circling the globe. Given that these diseases are largely air-, water-, or insect-borne and do not require sexual contact or blood-to-blood transmission, their potential for disaster is much greater than that of AIDS. Some of these epidemics are new. However, many are actually old diseases that modern medicine believed had been eradicated. Tuberculosis, the greatest killer during the first half of this century and possibly all time, has reemerged in new multiple-drug resistant (MDR) form. It currently claims three million lives annually and is the number one cause of death in the world today. In one California high school this year, a single 16-year-old girl infected 292 of her classmates (representing 23 percent of the student body) before her TB was diagnosed. New strains of cholera, yellow fever, malaria, and many others have also appeared for which there is no effective medical treatment. In Africa, Marburg and Ebola viruses have caused devastating epidemics in recent years. In one outbreak in Zaire, thirteen of seventeen doctors and nurses died while treating the disease. In the United States, deaths linked to hantaviruses carried by rodents have spread from the desert Southwest to the East Coast, and new virulent life-threatening strains of common bacteria have emerged, including a "flesh-eating" form of *streptococcus*. In the *Lancet*, the leading medical journal in England, several bacteriologists warned that the spread of AIDS, TB, and the new diseases constituted "the greatest health disaster since the bubonic plague."

Such warnings do not even consider the effects of environmental imbalance. The worldwide decline of songbirds and frogs, for example, could lead to a catastrophic proliferation of mosquitoes, fleas, and other insects that serve as vectors for the spread of viral and bacterial disease in humans. The introduction of new genetically engineered fruits and vegetables will inevitably lead to the emergence of new drug-resistant strains of microorganisms and new plagues.

Like the fall of the Berlin Wall and the breakup of the Soviet Union, the collapse of modern medicine and its wonder drugs and vaccines has happened so suddenly that we cannot fully grasp changed circumstances and their implications. Older, more fixed ways of thinking still govern our conduct, though we understand the imperative for change. In this book, we do not address in detail all the new viral and bacterial diseases that are emerging as we enter the 21st century (see Table on p. 4). However, the dietary and lifestyle suggestions that we offer for AIDS will also generally help prevent—and in some cases relieve—these conditions. The key point is understanding the beneficial nature of disease. Viral and bacterial sicknesses are actually protecting us. These conditions are alerting us to imbalance and warding off more serious chronic diseases in the future. If treated in time—with natural methods—they often can be relieved.

We would like to thank our many associates over the years who have contributed to investigating the relationship between AIDS and diet, including Martha Cottrell, M.D., co-author of *AIDS, Macrobiotics, and Natural Immunity* (Japan Publications, 1990); Elinor M. Levy, Ph.D., J. C. Beldekas, Ph.D., and P. H. Black, M.D., from the Department of Microbiology of Boston University's School of Medicine who participated in the macrobiotic AIDS study; and Lawrence H. Kushi, Sc.D., assistant professor of epidemiology, University of Minnesota School of Public Health. We are grateful to Edward Esko, our colleague at the Kushi Institute, for the Foreword and to Gale Jack, Alex's wife, for copyediting.

Despite the grave threat that they pose, AIDS and other newly emerging plagues offer us the opportunity to self-reflect and turn the whole course of modern civilization in a more healthful and peaceful direction. Together, the macrobiotic and holistic community, the scientific and medical profession, governmental agencies, and ordinary individuals and families must find a way to heal the earth and ensure humanity's continued biological and spiritual evolution.

Michio Kushi and Alex Jack
Brookline, Massachusetts
September, 1994

12

1

Modern Civilization at the Crossroads

Modern technological civilization reached a height in the twentieth century. Automobiles, airplanes, space ships, telephones, radios, televisions, and computers—among many other discoveries and inventions—resulted in unparalleled material development and a higher standard of living than in any previous age. However, amid this phenomenal advance, the human race on this planet began to experience widespread chaos and disorder, including personal sickness and the spread of hatred, prejudice, and war. The rise of modern civilization has been accompanied by the decline of human life at all levels—the physical, mental, psychological, social, ideological, and spiritual. This deterioration is so extensive that the quality of human life has changed completely when compared to that of even one century ago.

As we enter the 21st century, modern civilization is unable to cope with the epidemic spread of heart disease, cancer, mental and psychological illness, AIDS, and newly emerging infectious diseases. Nor has it been able to deal effectively with the decline of the family, loss of traditional values, increasing crime and social disorder, environmental pollution, and war. With the end of the Cold War between the United States and Soviet Union, the threat of global thermonuclear conflict has greatly decreased. However, the spread of nuclear weapons and technologies to smaller, more volatile states has increased, and the collapse of power blocs and states has resulted in widespread chaos and disorder.

Rather than being healthy, sound, and positive, civilization is defensive, protective, and negative. Advances in communication and transportation have contributed to uniting different continents, races, cultures, and customs, and may be considered relatively positive and unifying. But many other facets of modern life are polarizing and may be considered relatively negative and disruptive. These negative symptoms and factors include:

• Increasing numbers of hospitals and health-care facilities as well as spiralling medical costs and the growing number of health-care professionals to deal with the sharp rise in the rates of disease.

• Increasing complications in the judicial system, including the development of legal and informational technologies as well as the growing number of legal professionals, social service agencies, and correctional facilities to deal with the spread of crime, family abuse, and wild and anti-social behavior.

• Increasing mental health, self-development, and psychological training programs, and facilities as well as the expanding number of professionals to deal with increased mental and psychological disorders.

• Increasing insurance, investment, and mutual-security systems of various kinds, including public and private agencies and enterprises as well as government welfare and social systems, to deal with weakened social solidarity and the decline of individual and family ability to take responsibility for their own health and destiny.

• Increasing defense powers in the form of police at the domestic level and the military at the international level, including the development of nuclear weapons, chemical and biological weapons, and other weapons of mass destruction; espionage and counterespionage networks; and military-industrial alliances to deal with spreading distrust among people in communities, states, and nations.

• Increasing chemicalization and artificialization of the

drinking water and daily food supply; the development of the fast food, pharmaceutical, and biogenetic engineering industries; and the spread of organ transplants, test-tube births, and robots which are contributing to the weakening and sheltering effects of living in modern society and the possible eventual creation of an artificial species.

• Increasing belief systems including school and university education, the entertainment industry, the mass media, and many kinds of religious institutions to cope with prevailing human mental and spiritual instability.

These seven major aspects, along with many others, and the associated enterprises, industries, installations, and systems that service them, now compose the larger part of modern civilization. If humanity regained its natural health and developed a calm, peaceful, compassionate mind and heart, almost 90 percent of the activities associated with modern civilization would become unnecessary. However magnificent modern life appears to be in the realms of material wealth and technological sophistication, it is collapsing from sickness, negativity, and distrust on the inside. The time left to reverse this trend is running out.

The Spread of Degenerative Disease

Chronic diseases have spread rapidly through modern society. At the turn of the century, 1 in 25 people could expect to contract cancer. By 1950, it had risen to 1 in 8. Today, it is 1 in 3. Cardiovascular disease, including heart attack and stroke, affects 1 in 2 people. Arthritis afflicts 1 in 4 persons, mental or psychological illness 1 in 5, and diabetes 1 in 10. In comparison, AIDS affects 1 in 250 people in the United States. However, it is spreading rapidly. Among teenagers and young adults it is now the leading cause of death in some regions, doubling about every two to three years.

As for other viral and bacterial infections, carriers of the herpes virus may well exceed 30 percent of the current adult population in the United States, and cases of older venereal diseases, including syphilis and gonorrhea, are increasing rapidly. Tuberculosis is also rising dramatically. New types of viral diseases such as Epstein-Barr virus, which affects an individual's vitality and strength, are spreading rapidly.

The increasing rate of physical and mental disorders of modern civilization have coincided with changing dietary patterns and lifestyles. All other major factors, such as the motion of the earth, the movement of the solar system, and other celestial and terrestrial cycles have remained basically unchanged for thousands and perhaps millions of years. The seasons change, day and night cycle, and the ocean currents and tides ebb and flow pretty much the same as they have since human life first began on this planet. In comparison to these large, relatively constant natural factors, humanity's traditional way of eating and way of life have drastically changed, especially during the past several centuries coinciding with the industrial revolution. This change has continued to accelarate during the past seventy years, particularly after the Second World War. These dietary changes are so dramatic that humanity's biological, psychological, and spiritual condition has fundamentally altered, for better or worse, over the last several generations.

Lifestyle Changes

Among aspects of lifestyle that have also drastically changed in the modern era, the following artificial factors imposed on the human body and mind should also be considered in understanding the background to AIDS and the new plagues:

• Food and agricultural products have changed in quality from more whole and natural to more refined and partial. In the traditional way of eating, people received fiber, bran, protein, carbohydrates, fat, vitamins, minerals, enzymes, and other nutrients as part of a well balanced daily diet. Now they receive much of their nourishment in the form of pills, supplements, powders, and extracts and in food that has been fortified with additives or synthetic ingredients. In addition, most modern agricultural products are grown with chemical fertilizers, sprays, and pesticides and treated with additives, preservatives, and other artificial ingredients. Most recently, the irradiation and biogenetic engineering of food products has been introduced, further weakening the energy and nutrients of the foods we eat.

• Cooking sources have shifted from wood, charcoal, coal, gas, and other natural forms of heat to electricity and microwaves.

• Chemicals produced artificially have become a major part of daily life in food and drinks, cosmetics, cleaning materials, wrapping materials, carpeting, and building and decorative materials that compose exterior and interior environments.

• Clothing materials have shifted from more natural cotton or vegetable fibers to more synthetic materials used in everything from underwear to outerwear garments.

• Media have changed from simple materials made of paper such as books and newspapers to proportionately more use of radio, television, computers, satellites, and cable networks which now encircle the globe and produce a more unnatural, artificial electromagnetic environment.

• The modern synthetic living environment, especially in cities and other urban areas, has become densely fortified with concrete, metals, and insulation that separates us from the earth and sky and other natural forces that have supported the human race for millions of years.

• Inoculations and vaccinations, as well as the overuse of various types of drugs and medicines of which the majority are made of artificial chemical materials, have spread throughout society. These include the frequent use of antibiotics, X-rays, and routine operations to remove such vital glands and organs as the tonsils, appendix, ovaries, and uterus.

• To support these extensive changes of lifestyle, modern education has also shifted toward developing more technicians, experts, intellectuals, and specialists. Knowledge in general is limited only to certain areas of sensory measurement and intellectual development. Modern education has lost the view of humanity as a whole and has become separated from a rich heritage of natural health and well-being, intuitive consciousness and instinctive understanding.

• Family life has also changed from a natural bond of love and attraction based on biological and spiritual unity to a contractual agreement based on rights, concepts, and legal protection.

Dramatic lifestyle changes, including but certainly not limited to, the examples listed above, have extensively influenced modern life and consciousness, including prevailing physical and mental conditions. Without understanding the special characteristics of modern civilization that are shaping humanity's biological and spiritual evolution, we cannot discuss any issue affecting present-day human status including health and sickness, happiness and unhappiness, harmony and conflict, compassion and prejudice, peace and war.

The drastic changes of lifestyle and dietary patterns in modern civilization have contributed to the loss of humanity's natural adaptability to the natural planetary environment, including changes of climate, weather, temperature, humidity, wind, and other atmospheric and celestial influences. They have also accelerated the weakening of humanity's biological and spiritual quality, which is necessary for survival and for continued evolution.

In the case of viral and infectious diseases, there is a definite possibility that a large percentage of the world's population could perish within several decades. If the present trend continues without a revolutionary change of lifestyle and dietary practice and without deep reflection on the value of modern civilization and our personal way of life, human life as we have known it for thousands and possibly millions of years could come to an end.

Are there ways to prevent this vast disaster, or any measures to at least avoid the total destruction of modern civilization by controlling the speed and degree of viral infection, which is now spreading unchecked? To answer this question, we must discover why AIDS and related viral and bacterial actions have become active in recent years.

2

The Origin and Development of AIDS

The origin of AIDS is the subject of much study and controversy. Modern science and medicine—led by researchers at the Pasteur Institute and National Cancer Laboratory—views AIDS as primarily a viral disease and is devoting most of its time and energy to developing a vaccine to kill HIV and prevent its spread. Research indicates that AIDS emerged in Africa and shares an evolutionary connection with a primate disease. Investigators have found a genetic link between SIV—or Simian Immuodeficiency Virus, associated with monkeys—and HIV-1 and HIV-2—the two Human Immodeficiency Viruses. However, they cannot say yet whether the disease went from monkeys to humans or humans to monkeys. The microbes' earliest genetic line goes back several centuries, possibly a thousand years, but signs of virulence do not show up until the early 20th century and syptoms of illness did not appear until the late 1970s and early 1980s. Researchers do not know why AIDS suddenly manifested at this time. There are several major hypotheses including the following:

• HIV, a local infection, was spread globally by jet travel, international trade, and other features of modern transportation and communications.
• HIV initially spread through the American and Caribbean homosexual community, many members of which had developed susceptibility to viral infections as a result of over-

use of antibiotics for treatment of venereal disease or for heightened sexual enjoyment.

• SIV was transmitted to humans through a batch of contaminated polio vaccine prepared from infected monkey kidneys that was used widely in Africa in the 1960s.

These theories all point to the role that modern civilization—especially modern medicine—played in the spread of AIDS. But from the macrobiotic view, AIDS must be looked at on an even larger canvas. On the basis of environmental principles, we may hypothesis that in a traditional African setting, ancestors of SIV and HIV were relatively benign organisms that co-existed peacefully with animal and human populations for thousands of years. This is the general rule. In any ecosystem, multiple checks and balances create a system of homeostasis or balance.

Throughout history, most epidemics have been associated with social, cultural, or environmental factors that upset this delicate balance. For example, yellow fever—a major viral disease in recent centuries—is also associated with simian or monkey carriers. In hot, tropical countries, yellow fever was virtually unknown until modern times. It emerged following sweeping social and cultural changes in Latin America and Africa. Lands that had been traditionally used to grow grains, vegetables, tubers, and roots were colonized and turned over to the production of sugar, fruits, and other commodity crops. These foods attracted monkeys from the surrounding jungles. Aedes aegypti mosquitoes, in turn, feasted on the blood of infected monkeys, picked up the yellow fever virus, and passed it on to human beings. This is the ecological chain of transmission.

A similar process appears to underlie the emergence of AIDS. The regions in Central and West Africa where HIV-1 and 2 are believed to have originated were the site of former European colonies, including Zaire, Ivory Coast, Cameroons, Senegal, Gabon, and French Equatorial Africa. In addition to political and economic control over the last several hundred years, these areas were subject to the influx of legions of Western microbiologists, parasitologists, tropical physicians, and other scientists and public health officials who were apostles of the modern germ theory of disease and devoted to the sacred task of eradicating harmful microorganisms from the world.

From Brazzaville to Dakar, from Kinsasha to Nairobi, doctors and medical researchers served in the vanguard of the European colonial administration. In an article on "The Scientific Mission of the Institute Pasteur and the Colonial Experience" early in the century Calmette noted, "It is now the turn of the scientific experts to come onto the stage. . . . Their task is to draw up inventories of the natural resources of the conquered countries and to prepare the way for their expertise. These scientific experts are the geographers, engineers, and naturalists. Among the last, the microbiologists have a considerable role to play in protecting the colonies, their native collaborators, and their domestic animals against their most fearsome, because invisible, enemies."

Their methods resulted in uprooting millions of families, replacing traditional housing and farming practices with modern ones, and constructing mines, dams, highways, plantations, and the other colonial infrastructure that resulted in widespread ecological imbalance. In particular, traditional African farmlands were converted into vast plantations to produce sugar, cocoa, coffee, bananas, and other single commodity crops. The end result was an environmental catastrophe that set the stage for an endless cycle of poverty, hunger, starvation, drought, desertification, and disease.

After World War II, colonialism in Africa declined and political independence was attained. However, the economic pattern and effects of social dislocation continued. To deal with recurrent famines and epidemics, the United Nations mounted international relief efforts and private charities distributed millions of tons of infant formula, powdered milk, white flour, and canned food. Further, people living in Africa—as elsewhere around the world where a similar process was underway—were subjected to mass inoculations, antibiotics, and other drugs and medical procedures. In the short run, these measures helped saved millions of people suffering from acute infection and malnutrition. However, in the long run they weakened peoples' natural immunity to disease. In this setting, natural selection favored the evolution of virulent microbes that were resistant to vaccines, antibiotics, and drugs. The result has been a wave of infectious disease, including malaria, sleeping sickness, river blindness, hookworm, and—most lethally—AIDS.

In Africa, modernization (especially overgrazing by livestock and monoculture) created a legacy of unemployment, poverty, hunger, and sprawling urbanization as displaced farmers and their families flocked to cities and slums. "During the 1960s and 1970s extensive migrations occurred from rural areas in central and east Africa because of socioeconomic problems," biologist Paul Ewald explains in *Evolution of Infectious Diseases.* "This mobility in response to economic forces was partly a legacy of the colonial period, during which a migrant labor force developed in response to centralization of jobs. When agricultural options deteriorated, men left the agricultural areas to obtain industrial jobs. The large populations of men without families created a market for sexual commerce, drawing young women from rural into urban areas . . . " Amid this ecological and social imbalance, prostitution—both female and male—served as the primary vector for the transmission of the AIDS virus.

Briefly, the emerging ecological theory of infectious disease, including AIDS, is that clearing land for cattle pasture, sugar plantations, mining, logging, or urban development disrupts the local environment, favoring the emergence of microbes that are benign in a natural setting but that are virulent when natural checks and balances are eliminated or altered. Then as a result of international jet travel and trade, these microorganisms are swiftly transported to far distant climes and environments where they have no natural predators. In this way, new, extremely dangerous microorganisms can quickly spread around the world. In India, for example, Kyasanur Forest disease (KFD), a severe hemorrhagic disease, first appeared in the mid-1950s. Initially it affected monkeys and then spread into the human population. A generation ago, scientists would have declared the KFD virus a mutant organism that had arisen randomly and that had to be destroyed by any means necessary. Today, the approach is more sophisticated. "Ecological factors, including deforestation, cattle grazing, and an increased opportunity for tick density were probably responsible for the appearance of this disease, which has persisted as an endemic infection since that time," writes Thomas Monath in *Emerging Viruses*, an anthology of essays by current viral researchers. "The virus was probably circulating silently in ticks and rodent hosts; ecological changes provided an opportunity for amplified transmission, and human encroachment in this altered environment led to the emergence of epidemic disease." Social, cultural, and environmental measures will be more important in reversing this epidemic than medical treatment.

In Central and South America, the rain forests are being felled for timber, livestock production, mining, and ranching. The environmental movement has focused on how this is contributing to global warming by increasing the buildup of carbon dioxide in the atmosphere. An equally dangerous consequence of the loss of the tropical rain forests and biodiversity is the effect on microorganisms. Following ecological imbalance, selective forces may favor more virulent strains of microbes, which may emerge and disseminate around the world. In an essay "Global Change and Epidemiology" in *Emerging Viruses*, Thomas E. Lovejoy notes that populations of North American migratory birds that hibernate in the tropical forests have declined dramatically in the last decade. "This may occasionally upset the average bird watcher, but what does it mean to the rest of us? It turns out that most of those migratory passerines are very dependent on insect populations at the time they are raising young and are a major evolutionary influence on insect behavior and ecology. So even something as far fetched as conversion of Central American forest to cattle pasture could, in the end, have a major impact on the way viruses and other pathogens associated with birds or insects might behave in North America."

Increasingly ecology is seen as the key to understanding the development of animal and human epidemics. "Introduction of viruses into the human population is often the result of human activities, such as agriculture, that, cause changes in natural environment," explains Stephen S. Morse, a virologist at Rockefeller University, in *Emerging Viruses*. He shows, for example, that herbicides introduced into the Latin American pampas led to the rise of Argentine hemorrhagic fever beginning in 1960. The chemical sprays altered the ecology and led to the creation of a new mouse which was the carrier of the deadly virus.

Medically-Caused Infection

In *Evolution of Infectious Disease*, Paul Ewald applies evolutionary principles to the entire scope of modern medical treatment and comes to the paradoxical conclusion that many scientific strategies to combat infectious disease—such as hospitalization, vaccination, and antibiotics—may actually be increasing the incidence of disease. He shows that the virulence of potentially harmful microorganisms rapidly increases in a clinical setting and that many vaccines and drugs are counterproductive. By killing off the milder strains of microbes, they strengthen the stronger ones, which are then able to multiply better, spread more rapidly, and cause more serious damage. He cites current statistics showing that 1 in 20 patients in the United States—and 1 in 7 intensive care patients—acquires an infection in the hospital; one third of all pneumonia is acquired in the hospital, and one third of all these cases die; and hospital-acquired infection now ranks among the ten leading causes of death in modern society. Increasingly, he explains, hospital-caused infections are untreatable because the clinical setting favors the rapid evolution of drug-resistant species of microorganisms, and for many conditions, such as tuberculosis, there is currently no effective remedy.

"The present efforts to control infectious diseases generally do not involve assessment of evolutionary stability," he explains. "Rather, researchers focus on vulnerable aspects of a pathogen, such as biochemical components that can be used in a vaccine . . . If the individuals in a pathogen species always wore the same uniform, identifying and destroying them would be as easy as it was with smallpox. But most parasites practice guerrilla warfare . . . vaccines generated against sexually reproducing parasites like malaria, or mutation-prone viruses like HIV and influenza can be expected to provide partial and unstable solutions. Vaccination has already nullified easy adversaries. We are now left with the more wily ones, which probably will evade our vaccination efforts by changing their coats."

Rather than mass, multiple, broad-based vaccination campaigns to eradicate harmful microbes, Ewald suggests that we "use our knowledge about them to make them evolve into less dangerous organisms." Many current vaccines, he suggests, are unsafe and ineffective. In addition to occasionally causing "severe damage to those it is supposed to protect," the whooping cough vaccine, for example, produces increased virulence. If new vaccines do not take natural selection and the survival of the fittest into account, he concludes, "our vaccination efforts may backfire. We may be introducing large numbers of benign organisms into environments that will favor their evolutionary transformation into dangerous organisms."

Abuse of Antibiotics

Initially, penicillin and other antibiotics proved to be extremely effective, saving the lives of millions of people who otherwise would have died. However, the euphoria surrounding these "miracle drugs" quickly began to fade. Streptomycin almost completely lost its effectiveness after two months of use, especially on pulmonary tuberculosis. It also left many patients deaf or permanently dizzy. However, because the life-saving benefits still clearly outweighed the drawbacks, postwar physicians continued to prescribe strong drugs like these, and they became the treatment of choice for most acute conditions. Within several decades, they began to be used prophylactically to prevent future infection, as well as remedially to treat existing disease, and antibiotics were routinely added to lifestock feed, over-the-counter pharmaceuticals, cosmetics, and other non-prescription products.

In the United States, 240 million doses of antibiotics are prescribed every year, almost one per person. One of every three hospital patients receives an antibiotic, and physicians routinely administer antibiotics for everything from the common cold to pneumonia. Of course, colds are virally, not bacterially, associated, and antibiotics have no inhibitory effect. Nevertheless, because their patients demand strong medication, doctors acquiesce, though their use is contraindicated in many cases. Altogether, medical use accounts for 60 percent of antibiotic use. The other 40 percent is used in lifestock feed. By 1980, 75 percent of all cattle in the United States received antibiotics, 90 pecent of swine and veal calves, 50 percent of sheep, and nearly 100 percent of chickens and poultry. The drugs not only were used to prevent infection but to fatten up the animals and ensure maximum growth—and thus profits.

In recent years, research has shown that antibiotics can interfere with the production of red blood cells, the metabolism of vitamin B-12, and kill benign or beneficial bacteria in the intestines that synthesize Vitamin K, biotin, riboflavin, panthothenate, and pyridoxine. These nutrients are all associated with proper immune function and protection against disease. Side-effects associated with antibiotic use and misuse include diarrhea, rashes, fever, allergic reactions, hemolytic anemia, bleeding, bone marrow toxicity, and disorders of the kidneys, liver, and central nervous system. The spectacular spread of *candida albicans* and other acute infections has been associated with chronic antibiotic use that has disrupted the normal homeostasis in the digestive system and enabled the selection of pathogenic strains of yeast, fungi, bacilli, and other microorganisms.

"The sheer magnitude of this assault [the creation of new diseases by antibiotic-resistant microbes] is staggering," concludes Marc Lappé in his book *When Antibiotics Fail: Restoring the Ecology of the Body.* "For four decades now, we have thrown hundreds of tons of antibiotics against our Hollywood imagination of microscopic enemies. In the process we have sown seeds for a whole new array of actual germs and diseases. . . . We favor simple technological fixes for complex disease entities, while our medical complex fosters a near-sighted one-germ, one-chemical mentality. Together, these positions contribute to a world view that encourages the proliferation of new chemotherapeutic agents, and in turn, the proliferation of new disease entitles. . . . The answer clearly does not consist of throwing more troops into a losing battle."

Reverse Evolution

There may be another dimension to the origin of AIDS that modern science and medicine have not considered. AIDS—in some cases—may be self-caused. It may arise as a result of reverse evolution, or the decomposition of blood cells, lymph cells, and other normal body cells into bacteria, viruses, DNA, and other more primitive forms of life. During a period of over 3 billion years of planetary evolution, biological transformation proceeded from elements and compounds to viruses, from viruses to bacteria, from bacteria to single-cell organisms, from single-cell organisms to multi-cellular organisms, from multi-cellular organisms to simple skeletal organisms, from simple skeletal organisms to complex skeletal organisms, and from complex skeletal organisms to present human beings.

From this perspective, we can understand that biological degeneration represents a reversal of the evolutionary process. When human beings stop eating food in harmony with nature—predominantly whole cereal grains and cooked vegetables as their main food—they can no longer adapt to their changing environment and begin to lose their human condition and quality.

Biological degeneration can transform multi-cellular organisms to single-cell organisms, and single-cell organisms may revert back to bacteria and viruses. In the human body, individual cells that are not properly nourished can degenerate into more primitive stages of life. Such cell degeneration would possibly occur more easily in less-developed cells such as blood cells, especially white-blood cells and reproductive follicles, than in well-developed body cells.

27

Such degeneration could arise if the body's internal environment reproduced environmental conditions similar to the primordial conditions of the earth when bacteria and viruses flourished. If the blood, lymph, body fluid, and interior of the intestines, as well as reproductive organs, increase their content of fatty acids, sulfur compounds, uric acid, ammonium compounds, methane gas and other gaseous conditions, and decrease their content of minerals, white-blood cells and other more primitive human cells may weaken and degenerate into bacteria and viruses. In other words, AIDS may not in all cases be transmitted virally from the outside through sexual or other contact with someone who is infected. AIDS may arise, in some cases, internally from the long-time degenerative effects of dietary and environmental imbalance. We must emphasize that this hypothesis—based on the macrobiotic understanding of the order of nature—requires further study. It may explain, however, why AIDS-related symptoms have appeared in some individuals who have not been exposed to HIV-1 or HIV-2 through sexual contact or other known means of transmission.

In the late 19th century, Louis Pasteur, the father of microbiology and the germ theory of disease, observed that microorganisms commonly change their properties, including their virulence, within an organism and under varying environmental conditions. Early in this century, medical researchers began to study the fermentative, morphological, and other properties of microorganisms and reported that microbes could transform into one another. In the *Journal of Infectious Diseases* early in the century, E. C. Rosenow of the Memorial Institute for Infectious Diseases in Chicago reported that in laboratory experiments *pneumococci* (the microbes associated with pneumonia) could be transmuted into *streptococci* (the microbes associated with strep infections). His conclusion that nutritional and environmental factors may cause microorganisms to change or transmute into pathogenic species within the body without stimulus or entry from outside flew in the face of scientific theory regarding the fixity of species and hence was never seriously considered.

More recently, in *Virus Hunting: AIDS, Cancer, and the*

Human Retrovirus, Dr. Robert Gallo, the co-discoverer of HIV, refers to a similar theory, "Some scientists have speculated that in a weird case of reverse evoluton, viruses are descended from more complex parasites, adapting by shedding their ingredients to the barest form capable of survival . . . "

The mechanism of this process, of course, is unclear. The mitochondrion—a microscopic body found in the cells of almost all living organisms and containing enzymes responsible for the conversion of food to usable energy—may revert to a bacterium under certain circumstances. A bacterium, in turn, may revert to a virus. Current research into viroids, prions, plasmids, and microorganisms that are smaller than viruses could also throw light onto this subject.

Even if future research shows that such degeneration of primitive cells does not occur within the body, the acid condition of the body's internal environment which simulates the primordial earth could easily receive, activate, and spread harmful microorganisms. HIV-1 and HIV-2, as we have seen, may have existed in benign or dormant form as part of a stable natural environment from the beginning of biological evolution until very recently. Following modification or destruction of their natural environment, these microbes may have evolved into virulent organisms capable of spreading rapidly within the human population. HIV-1 appears to be more prevalent in people who have consumed various acid-producing foods but at the same time including animal sources such as meat, dairy food, and so on in their diet. HIV-2 appears to be more common in people who have been consuming almost exclusively vegetable sources of acid-producing food including excessive consumption of sugar, chocolate, fruit, vegetable oils, and the like, without much animal food.

According to recent scientific observation, the AIDS virus appears to be exceptionally capable of hiding in the various parts of the human system. These parts include intestinal tissues, cervical tissues, the interior of the uterus and vagina, as well as the male reproductive organs. Macrophages, which are special sacks inside large cells, appear to become laden with AIDS viruses and carry them to rectal cells, cervical cells, vaginal fluids and semen. If the environment of these cells and fluids changes and becomes more suitable for the activity of viruses, they will be released and become more active. Furthermore, it appears that these viruses overcoat their protein surface with sugar molecules which protect the surface of the viruses from antibodies activated by the body's immune function. This scientific observation suggest that viruses may be produced through decomposition of large cells. Regardless, dietary habits rich in acid-producing factors and overconsumption of foods rich in simple sugars appear to preserve, protect, and activate AIDS viruses. As noted above, a weakened internal environment is produced by various extreme and undesirable factors of modern life, especially improper dietary habits which result in more fat, mucus, and acidic conditions in the blood and body fluid, the intestines, and the reproductive organs. Therefore, return to a more balanced way of life and dietary practice is essential to prevent AIDS and other infectious and communicable diseases.

3

Natural Immunity
to Disease

There are many natural limitations or boundaries that serve to maintain existence and achieve continuous development of humanity on this planet. From an ecological view, we can easily see that human beings living in modern society have exceeded natural limitations and lack comprehensive awareness of the factors and conditions necessary for continued existence. Because viral and bacterial infection—or natural immune deficiency—is a biological phenomenon, not a social phenomenon such as war or group violence, there must be some human factors violating this biological order.

Factors supporting the biological status of humanity can be divided into two broad groups: 1) external environment and stimuli and 2) internal environment and stimuli. In turn, each of these groups can be divided into two subgroups: 1) natural and 2) human-made:

• **Natural external factors and stimuli:** Movement of the universe, galaxies and solar systems, and the planet earth. Natural atmospheric and oceanic influences; seasonal and climatic changes including temperature, humidity, and pressures; and other natural influences.
• **Human-made external factors and stimuli:** Civilizational and cultural influence, social structures and conditions,

economical and community influences, human relations, oc-
cupational and professional stimuli, technological and artificial influences, transportation and communications stimuli,
and all other human-made surroundings and their stimuli.
  • **Natural internal environmental factors and stimuli:**
The various systems and functions of the body and mind including the digestive system, the circulatory system, the nervous system, the excretory system, the skeletal and muscular
system, the meridians or pathways of natural electromagnetic
energy, and all other organs, glands, and channels associated
with our physical, mental, and spiritual constitution. The
food, drink, waves, rays, and other incoming substances and
vibrations that are received, digested, absorbed, transmuted,
and discharged by the above systems and functions.
  • **Human-made internal environmental factors and
stimuli:** Physical, mental, psychological, spiritual, and social
images, thoughts, actions, influences, and other impulses and
movements generated from within and governed by our
higher consciousness centers or autonomic nervous system.

  What the human body takes in from the external environment changes and is transformed into the internal environment. Energies coming from the universe and atmosphere are
running through meridians—channels of electromagnetic energy in the body—and are distributed to every cell. Conscious
images are also carried through the meridians and charge
each cell. What we eat and drink forms our cells and nourishes them with various nutrients and natural electromagnetic
energy. This nourishment is carried through the digestive and
circulatory systems and is distributed to all cells.
  This internal environment, though its sources come from
outside in the external environment, is largely shaped and
controlled by personal freedom. What kind of food, how it is
prepared, and how much is consumed all depend on personal
choice. Except during times of extreme scarcity or other unu-
sual conditions, free consciousness is exercised completely in
respect to what we eat and drink. Accordingly, the internal
environment differs among individual people, while external
environmental stimuli are more or less common to everyone.

Among the factors supporting humanity on this planet, individual differences—physical, mental, spiritual, and social—are largely dependent upon factors producing the internal environment, especially what we eat and drink daily, upon which everyone exercises his or her free consciousness. Accordingly, to solve the problem of why a certain person can be easily infected by an infectious virus or bacterium, while another person is not easily affected, we have to review differences in dietary practice. Of course, we must consider whether the way of eating in any given environment is suitable for existence and development under the prevailing external conditions and stimuli. Certain dietary practices may be more suitable than others, while others may not be suitable for sustaining and supporting life at all.

The macrobiotic view of dietary practice, which considers food as a natural means of adapting, maintaining, and developing humanity, observes the following principles:

• Respect for traditional dietary practices followed by many generations in a given area because these have been securing, maintaining, and developing humanity in that particular natural setting for thousands of years.

• Respect for the traditional way of preparation and cooking which has been exercised for centuries in a particular natural environment for similar reasons.

• Respect for the food, ways of natural preparation, and cooking that developed in natural environments and climates similar to our own. This concept enables us to avoid exceeding natural limitations, which are violated when we adopt too much food or drink, ways of preparation, or cooking methods from environments different or opposite to our own.

If we review modern dietary practice, we find that the above principles are constantly violated. Since the 1940s and 1950s, when "miracle drugs" were first introduced, food quality has steadily deteriorated. The quality of chocolate, sugar, fruit, chicken, meat and other foods associated with infectious disease has greatly declined, giving rise to stronger microorganisms and new strains of disease. Violations may be summarized briefly as follows:

- Abandonment of whole food through refining, milling, and other processing techniques.
- Adoption of artificial, chemicalized agriculture and abandonment of naturally and organically grown food.
- Overconsumption of simple sugars with a decrease in the consumption of complex sugars.
- Overconsumption of animal-quality protein with decreased consumption of vegetable-quality protein.
- Overconsumption of saturated fat, largely of animal quality, and decreased consumption of unsaturated fat of vegetable quality.
- Lack of natural vitamins resulting from the increased refinement of naturally grown products and the waste of edible and traditionally consumed parts of vegetable foods.
- Lack of consumption of natural dietary fiber due to food processing, including refining and milling.
- Disorderly consumption of minerals by the refining of salts and other food products, as well as the overuse of chemical fertilizers, insecticides, preservatives, and colorings.
- Disorderly use of natural enzymes by artificially altering traditional methods of food processing, including fermentation and pickling.
- Shift from family cooking to the industrial and commercial preparation of food, which also standardizes the way of eating and preparation regardless of regional, seasonal, climatic, and personal differences.
- Introduction of hybridized, irradiated, genetically-engineered, and other artificially produced food.

To change dietary practice in a more healthy direction, one that is in harmony with the natural environment, the following guidelines may be observed:

- Food should be more naturally and organically grown, avoiding or minimizing various artificial chemicals in production, cultivation, and processing.
- The majority of food is to be grown and produced in the same climatic and geographical region where the people who eat it are living. In the event transportation of food from

a distance is necessary, this food should come from similar climatic belts and natural environments.

• Food is to be consumed in whole form as much as possible except for the inedible portion which may be set aside. Refining of food is to be avoided. Whole food secures more balance of nutrients, including fiber, minerals, vitamins, and other necessary components, than food that is processed or consumed in parts.

• The majority of food is to be vegetable quality rather than animal quality, except for dietary practice in the poorer regions of the world or in cold climates in temperate or polar regions. The main source of food is to originate from the plant kingdom.

• Animal food, if consumed, is to be lower in hard, saturated fat and cholesterol, and amount to less than 15 percent of total daily food consumption. In polar or colder regions the percentage may be slightly higher.

• Carbohydrates are to be taken more in the form of complex sugars (such as those found in whole cereal grains) rather than simple sugars (such as those found in dairy products, fruits, and sweeteners).

• Protein is to come from more vegetable and plant sources and less from animal sources.

• Fat should come more from vegetable and plant sources and be more unsaturated in quality and less from animal sources and be less saturated in quality.

• Minerals should be consumed as a part of whole-food items. In addition, naturally processed unrefined sea salt, which consists of many trace minerals beside sodium chloride, should be used in cooking.

• Vitamins should be consumed as a part of whole foods and not be taken separately as a supplement.

• Enzymes should be consumed as a part of daily foods including fermented and pickled food and not be taken separately as an enzyme supplement.

• Beverages are based upon natural spring or well water and nonstimulant, nonaromatic beverages traditionally and widely used.

Guidelines for Food Preparation

In processing food from its natural form to an edible form, we observe methods traditionally practiced over centuries using more natural energies. The natural energies applied to food processing include: drying under the sun or in the shade without direct exposure to solar energy; soaking in natural water; applying pressure and weight; pickling with sea salt; smoking by wood fire or charcoal; fermenting under natural atmospheric conditions, for hours, days, weeks, months, and in some cases several years depending on the kinds of food products and the strength desired; milling by motion of natural stone or hardwood; pressing with comparatively low temperatures; cooking with natural water and fire made of wood, charcoal, or gas; and roasting slowly with a moderate fire produced by wood, charcoal, or gas.

These natural food-processing methods are found in most parts of the world and have been perfected over the centuries by many traditional civilizations and cultures. They all avoid the use of destructive, explosive energies and quick energetic and molecular change of food components such as we find in modern food processing techniques and in electrical and microwave cooking. Moderate transformation of food quality using more natural forces is the essential principle of traditional, healthy, natural food processing. In order to maintain a food's integrity—including its genuine energy, quality, and balance of nutrients—traditional methods of food processing are far superior to quick processing techniques utilizing high technology and applying highly unnatural, violent forces.

Considering the above guidelines, it is recommended that the actual dietary practice in the temperate regions of the world—including most of North America, Europe, Russia, China, the Far East, Australia, and temperate parts of Africa and Latin America—be as follows for people in usual good health.

Daily Dietary Recommendations

1. Whole cereal grains. At least 50 percent by weight of every meal is recommended to include cooked, organically grown, whole cereal grains prepared in a variety of ways. Whole cereal grains include brown rice, barley, millet, oats, corn, rye, wheat, and buckwheat. A small portion of this amount may consist of noodles or pasta, unyeasted whole grain breads, and other partially processed whole cereal grains.

2. Soups. Approximately 5 to 10 percent of your daily food intake may include soup made with vegetables, sea vegetables (wakame or kombu), grains or beans. Seasonings are usually miso (fermented soybean paste) or shoyu (natural soy sauce). The flavor should not be too salty.

3. Vegetables. About 20 to 30 percent of daily intake may include local and organically grown vegetables. Preferably, the majority are cooked in various styles (e.g., sautéed with a small amount of sesame or corn oil, steamed, boiled and sometimes prepared using shoyu or light sea salt as a seasoning). A small portion may be eaten as raw salad. Pickled vegetables without spice may also be used daily in small volume.

Vegetables for daily use include green cabbage, kale, broccoli, cauliflower, collards, pumpkin, watercress, Chinese cabbage, bok choy, dandelion, mustard greens, daikon greens, scallion, onions, daikon, turnips, acorn squash, butternut squash, buttercup squash, burdock, carrots, and other seasonally grown varieties.

Avoid potatoes (including sweet potatoes and yams), tomatoes, eggplant, peppers, asparagus, spinach, beets, zucchini, and avocado for regular use. Mayonnaise and other oily, greasy, or fatty dressings should be avoided.

4. Beans and Sea Vegetables. Approximately 5 to 10 percent of our daily diet includes cooked beans and sea vegetables. The most suitable beans for regular use are azuki beans, chickpeas, and lentils. Other beans may be used on occasion. Bean products such as tofu, tempeh, and natto can also be used. Sea vegetables such as nori, wakame, kombu, hijiki, arame, dulse, agar-agar, and Irish moss may be prepared in small volume in a variety of ways. They can be cooked with beans or vegetables, used in soups, or served separately as side dishes, flavored with a moderate amount of shoyu, sea salt, brown rice vinegar, umeboshi plum, and others.

5. Occasional Foods. If needed or desired, one to three times per week, approximately 5 to 10 percent of that day's consumption of food can include fresh white-meat fish such as flounder, sole, cod, carp, halibut or trout.

Fruit or fruit desserts, including fresh, dried, and cooked fruits, may also be served two or three times a week. Local and organically grown fruits are preferred. If you live in a temperate climate, avoid tropical and semi-tropical fruit and eat, instead, temperate climate fruits such as apples, pears, plums, peaches, apricots, berries, and melons. Frequent use of fruit juice is not advisable. However, occasional consumption in warmer weather may be appropriate depending on your health.

Lightly roasted nuts and seeds such as pumpkin, sesame, and sunflower seeds, peanuts, walnuts, and pecans may be enjoyed as a snack.

Rice syrup, barley malt, and amasake (a sweet rice beverage) may be used as a sweetener; brown rice vinegar or umeboshi vinegar may be used occasionally for a sour taste.

6. Beverages. Recommended daily beverages include roasted bancha twig tea, stem tea, roasted brown rice tea, roasted barley tea, dandelion tea, and cereal grain coffee. Any traditional tea that does not have an aromatic fragrance or a stimulating effect can be used. You may also drink a moderate amount of water (preferably spring or well water of good quality) but not iced.

7. Foods to Eliminate for Better Health. Meat, animal fat, eggs, poultry, dairy products (including butter, yogurt, ice cream, milk, and cheese), refined sugars, chocolate, molasses, honey, other simple sugars and foods treated with them, and vanilla.

Tropical or semi-tropical fruits and fruit juices, soda, artificial drinks and beverages, coffee, colored tea, and all aromatic stimulating teas such as mint or peppermint tea.

All artificially colored, preserved, sprayed or chemically treated foods. All refined and polished grains, flours, and their derivatives. Mass-produced industrialized food including all canned, frozen, and irradiated foods.

Hot spices, any aromatic stimulating food or food accessory, artificial vinegar, and strong alcoholic beverages.

8. Additional Suggestions. Cooking oil should be vegetable quality only. To improve your health, it is preferable to use only unrefined sesame or corn oil in moderate amounts.

• Salt should be naturally processed sea salt. Traditional, non-chemicalized shoyu and miso may also be used as seasonings.

• Recommended condiments include: gomashio (16-18 parts roasted sesame seeds to 1 part roasted sea salt); sea-vegetable powder (kelp, kombu, wakame, and other sea vegetables); sesame sea-vegetable powder; umeboshi plums; tekka; shoyu (moderate use, use only in cooking for mild flavoring); pickles (made using bran, miso, shoyu, salt), sauerkraut.

• You may have meals regularly, 2-3 times per day, as much as you want, provided the proportion is correct and chewing is thorough. Avoid eating for approximately 3 hours before sleeping.

9. The Importance of Cooking. Proper cooking is very important for health. Everyone should learn to cook either by attending classes or studying under with an experienced macrobiotic cook. The recipes included in macrobiotic cookbooks may also be used in planning your meals.

These dietary recommendations not only satisfy modern nutritional requirements but they are also effective in helping to prevent major degenerative diseases including heart disease, hypertension, cancer, allergies, arthritis, diabetes, hypoglycemia, and many others, as well as reproductive and gynecological problems and various types of mental, psychological, and emotional instability. For a summary of 265 scientific and medical studies showing the physical, mental, and environmental benefits of macrobiotics and natural foods, please see *Let Food Be Thy Medicine*, by Alex Jack, One Peaceful World Press.

Tropical and Semitropical Guidelines

Traditionally, in South Asia, Southeast Asia, Africa, Central and South America, and other tropical and semitropical regions, people have been eating cooked whole cereal grains as principal food. The grain, including long-grain rice, basmati rice, sorghum, and others, is complemented with vegetables, as well as soup and broth, beans and sea vegetables, and other categories of food in the Standard Macrobiotic Diet.

Proportions of foods, cooking styles, seasoning, and other factors may differ from standard cooking in temperate regions. For example, for those in usual good health, the amount of vegetables, fresh raw salad, and fruit may be slightly higher; steaming, stir-frying, braising, and other lighter cooking methods may be used more frequently, including boiling of grain rather than pressure-cooking; and less salt, miso, shoyu, or lighter miso and other seasonings may be used. However, in a hot and humid climate, a salty taste may often be more required than in a temperate climate.

In addition to whole grains, some cultures and island societies have traditionally consumed cassava, taro, yams, sweet potatoes, and other roots and tubers as staple food. In such cases, these may be included in the grain category as the principal source of complex carbohydrates.

In addition to fish and seafood, a small volume of wild animals, birds, and insects may be eaten if traditionally prepared and commonly consumed. Also a small volume of spices, herbs, and aromatic, fragrant beverages may be taken on occasion to help offset the high heat and humidity.

For a list of typical foods in tropical and semitropical regions, as well as guidelines for polar and semipolar regions, please see *Standard Macrobiotic Diet* by Michio Kushi, One Peaceful World Press. Persons with AIDS or those who test positive for HIV in either a temperate or tropical climate should observe the dietary recommendations listed below in Chapter 9.

Understanding Microorganisms

Microorganisms are everywhere. They are all around us, they are inside of us, they are on us. Microbes inhabit every part of our bodies. Without them we could not live. They help synthesize important nutrients and protect us from various illnesses. Altogether the human body harbors an estimated 100 trillion microorganisms, nearly all of which are beneficial.

In the mid-1950s, at the height of the miracle drug era, René Dubos, one of the pioneers in modern biochemistry and developer of antibiotics, called for a reappraisal of the germ theory of disease and modern medicine's entire strategy of treatment. In identifying factors that can lower resistance and bring on sickness, Dubos explained in a lead article in *Scientific-American,* "The stimulus may be a fever of unrelated origin, excessive irradiation, certain types of surgery, menstruation or improper food." Susceptibility to infection, Dubos went on to state, is linked to physiology and the metabolic state. Scientists at his own laboratory at the Rockefeller Institute, he pointed out, "have shown that one can increase the susceptibility of mice to microbial disease by metabolic manipulations as simple as temporary deprivation of food, or feeding an unbalanced diet . . . Furthermore, resistance can be brought back to normal within two to three days by correcting the nutritional disorder."

Calling for a "a new look at the biological formulation of the germ theory," Dubos proposed that the whole nature of health and sickness must be looked at within an ecological context. Practically all common microbes, he stated, are ordinarily harmless, but are capable of producing disease when physiological circumstances are sufficiently disturbed. "These ubiquitous microbes rarely cause death, but they are certainly responsible for many ill-defined ailments—minor or severe—which constitute a large part of the miseries and 'disease' of everyday life. They establish a bridge between communicable and noncommunicable disease—a zone where presence of the microbe is the prerequisite but not the determinant of disease, a situation in which the fact of infection is less decisive in shaping the course of events than the physiological climate of the invaded body."

"[I]t is unlikly that antimicrobial drugs can control this aspect of the relationship between man and microbe," Dubos concluded. "What is most needed at the present time is some knowledge of the physiological and biochemical determinants of microbial diseases. For we cannot possibly hope to eliminate all the microbes that are potentially capable of causing harm to us. Most of them are an inescapable part of our environment."

The reason why viral and bacterial infections spread within a single body, after being transmitted from one body to another, is that the person or persons involved already have weakened natural immunity. Immune factors do not exist separately from comprehensive health conditions. Immune factors are the result of the healthy functioning of all major organs, glands, blood, lymphatic body fluids, hormones, digestive liquid and enzymes, together with sound skeletal, nervous, muscular, and skin functions of the entire body.

Strong immunity to disease—including protection against viral and bacterial infection—is a natural function of a healthy physical and mental human condition, and deficiency of natural immunity is the result of an unhealthy, degenerative human condition. Accordingly, any approach focusing exclusively on isolating a certain virus or bacterium cannot solve the problem of AIDS and related symptoms, though they may be affected temporarily by suppressing infectious agents. The solution lies within a comprehensive approach to recovering total health, including physical mental, and spiritual health and well-being. It is achieved by correcting modern lifestyles and dietary habits that are in violation of natural limits or natural order and by changing toward a more natural and healthy way of life and way of eating.

Natural Immune Function

The purpose of the human immune function is to maintain personal existence and to develop an individual's biological and spiritual quality under ever-changing environmental conditions. Natural immunity is the function most directly connected with exercising universal principles of natural order. It works constantly according to laws of attraction and repulsion. It also works with expansion and contraction, decomposition and composition, the process of evolution and the process of degeneration, and the process of forming and the process of decaying.

Human natural immunity includes the following functions:

• Adaptation to the environment
• Maintenance of existence
• Continuous biological and spiritual evolution, especially involving the quality and scope of consciousness.

To secure these functions, human natural immunity has an eight-fold constitution. This includes:

1. Intuition and Instinct. When a new factor is introduced into our environment, primary intuitive and instinctive judgment immediately act or react to this influence. They adapt to the new factor by enabling us to change ourselves, or by rejecting and avoiding the new factor. Intuitive and instinctive judgment are constantly at work in the selection of our place of residence, our partners and friends, our occupations and habits, and numerous occasions and conditions of daily life. Avoidance of danger, caution of abrupt, dramatic change, and seeking a middle way between extremes are all manifestations of intuitive and instinctive judgment. Without these functions, human life cannot be maintained and developed, and human identity would vanish.

2. Consciousness. Human consciousness includes the sensory, emotional, intellectual, social, and ideological levels. In the exercise of this consciousness, and levels work through the processes of discrimination, selection, and attraction or repulsion. For example, consciousness functions to make distinctions in the following ways: a) the sensory level distinguishes pleasure and pain, b) the emotional level distinguishes love and hate, c) the intellectual level distinguishes truth and error, d) the social level distinguishes justice and injustice, and e) the philosophical or spiritual level distinguishes freedom and necessity.

Through the exercise of this judgment, natural selection involving attraction or repulsion, and absorption or expulsion, are constantly being made for certain tendencies, objects, behaviors, or persons. As long as these levels of consciousness are working, extremes can be avoided without exposing us to danger.

3. **Autonomic Response.** In addition to the central nervous system, which mainly serves to produce and exercise consciousness, autonomic nerves—sympathetic and parasympathetic—function to react immediately to surrounding stimuli. Depending upon the kind of stimulus, sympathetic nerves control the immediate contraction of certain organs and glands as well as parts of the body. For an opposite type of stimulus, parasympathetic nerves produce an opposite reaction causing certain organs and glands to expand. For example, the pupil dilates in darkness and it contracts in bright light through this autonomic nerve response.

When the sympathetic nerve operates, the stomach expands and the connected sphincter contracts, while the parasympathetic nerve acts to contract the stomach and expand the sphincter. Through autonomic control, the necessary balance and harmony with the stimulus can be maintained for preserving and supporting the life of the organism.

4. **Body Surface Protection and Reaction.** For physical and chemical invasion and stimuli, the skin functions to protect the inner environment and reacts by contraction and expansion according to the nature of the stimuli. In cold temperature, for example, the skin becomes dry and shrinks, while in warmer temperature it becomes more moist and expands. When a physical shock is given to a certain part of the body surface, immediate reaction is experienced on the skin. More blood, especially white-blood cells and lymphatic liquid, gathers, often resulting in swelling of that portion of the skin. Further, slightly salty alkaline moisture secreted by sweat glands protects the body from invasion of acid poison. The body surface also acts to expel toxins and unnecessary ener-

gies from the inside of the body to the surface. These discharges often appear as various types of skin disease and discolorations, as well as skin cancer.

5. **Internal Liquid Protection.** Through digestive functions, alkaline liquid and acid liquid are alternatively secreted in the body in the form of digestive liquids. First food is subjected to the action of saliva (alkaline) in the mouth. Then stomach liquid (acid) is secreted, followed by liver and gallbladder biles and pancreatic juice (alkaline). Finally, metabolized foodstuffs are readied for absorption in the small intestine by intestinal juice (acid). These digestive liquids minimize and neutralize poisonous chemical and biological factors, including the undesirable action of microorganisms, in addition to normal food decomposition and digestive functions. Proper chewing facilitates the immune process. The more we chew, the more saliva is produced. Saliva accelerates these protective functions, enhancing other digestive secretions and related nervous activities. The *Journal of the American Dental Association* reported that human saliva prevented the AIDS virus from infecting lymphocytes and contained substances that kill bacteria and fungi.

Further, immunoglobulin A (IGA) existing in the internal fluids secreted throughout the digestive system (and in other systems such as the reproductive system) as well as on intercellular fluids can act as a protective agent from poisonous substances that have entered from outside the body or that have been produced inside the body. The protective functions of IGA in the mouth cavity together with saliva and in the wall surface around and in between numerous villi in the small intestine are especially active in neutralizing and minimizing the undesirable activities of viruses, bacteria, and other microorganisms.

6. **Blood and Intercellular Fluid Protection and Reaction.** Within the bloodstream, there are constant balancing mechanisms and buffer actions to neutralize strong toxic acid compounds, changing them to weak acids through the mobilization of minerals in the body. These minerals are normally supplied in the daily diet, but if additional minerals are required for this buffer action, stored minerals are used. As a re-

sult, weakening of the bones often arises following the consumption of excessive amounts of acid-producing foods such as meat, dairy, and sugar. In children, this is the chief cause of tooth decay. In older people, chronic weakening of the bones from improper diet can lead to a potentially crippling condition known as osteoporosis.

Further, white-blood cells protect from undesirable viral and bacterial invasion. White-blood cells known as lymphocytes have various kinds of cells, such as B-cells and T-cells. These cells coordinate the maintenance of normal conditions by either neutralizing or harmonizing the poisonous effects of invading viruses or other microorganisms. Among their functions there are antagonistic-complemental relations constantly working as well-known helpers and suppressors. Among the group of T-cells, antagonistic-complemental relations between T4 cells and T8 cells are one of the balancing and harmonizing activities relating to undesirable viruses and microorganisms.

Because lymphocytes can exist within the body's intercellular fluids—that is, outside the bloodstream—these actions also arise within this location.

In addition, when foreign substances such as undesirable viruses or bacteria enter the blood and intercellular fluids, antagonistic and complementary factors can naturally be produced. These are called antibodies. The purpose of antigen production is to balance and harmonize foreign substances and maintain continuous body functions. Accordingly, the presence of antibodies can be an indication of the activity of undesirable viruses or other microorganisms within the individual.

7. Lymphatic Protection. After the blood and intercellular fluids nourish various body cells, they are collected in the lymph system. A great number of lymph nodes form a network throughout the body for cleaning undesirable wastes. If the collected fluids contain a great amount of undesirable poisonous wastes, various kinds of minerals are mobilized into the lymph nodes to make drastic action or cleaning. This action often results in the swelling of the lymph nodes. If such poisonous effects continue for some period, chronic swelling of lymph nodes and the spleen and ineffectiveness in the function of the lymphatic system arises as in the case of lymphoma.

In connection with this function, the surgical removal of some important lymph nodes such as the tonsils also directly contributes to the inefficiency of lymphatic functions and a general weakening of the natural immune system.

8. Cellular Protection. Each cell of the human body has its own protective function to maintain its identity and existence. Cell membranes act for direct protection from undesirable physical stimuli and chemical invasion. Firm bonding of several elements in DNA and RNA is not easily impaired unless the power of foreign substances and stimuli far exceeds the protective mechanism. Cell membranes and intercellular fluids also serve to protect the nucleus of the cell.

Each cell is constantly rejuvenated by the energy and nutrients that are being supplied through blood and intercellular fluids. Accordingly, if the quality of blood and intercellular fluids changes substantially, the quality of cells also inevitably changes. Such changes arise not only in the cell membrane and intercellular fluids, but also possibly in the nucleus of the cell.

These eight aspects of natural immunity do not function completely independently. Each acts to ensure its integrity, and yet all are interrelated and united as a whole. The decline of natural immunity—leading to AIDS or other immunedeficiency or infectious condition—is not the result of a sudden failure, defect, or ineffectiveness in one or more of these immune functions. It is the result of partial or total failure or decay of all of them, usually over a period of time.

The primary origin of natural immune deficiency is cloudiness in intuition and instinct. The decline of intuitive and instinctive judgment causes us to observe abnormal lifestyles and dietary practices that exceed the natural limitations of our environment, climate, constitution, or condition. Adopting imbalanced ways of life and eating, in turn, results in the further decay and weakening of other levels of the natural immune system.

While the primary origin of immune deficiency is the decline of intuitive-instinctive response, the biological cause of natural immunity is improper dietary habits. In other words, when intuitive-instinctive judgment is not exercised naturally in our daily eating, the decline of our natural immunity begins, and harmful viruses and bacteria in our environment can easily affect either some or all of the systems of the body.

Essentially, with AIDS the body—including blood, lymph, body cells, and immune cells—becomes progressively weaker from poor eating, and, as in other autoimmune disorders, the body begins to attack itself. At the cellular level, there is a deficiency of T4 cells, which produce antibodies to the virus. As a consequence, the virus continues to multiply, invading, devouring, and eventually killing the host.

"HIV infection may be an epiphenomenon of immune suppression rather than a necessary cause," Robert Root-Bernstein notes in *Rethinking AIDS*. "Immune suppression may predispose people to HIV infection (just as it predisposes them to other opportunistic infections) rather than resulting from such an infection."

Nutritional Factors

The energy and nutrients of the food we eat day to day creates, nourishes, and governs the quality and volume of blood and intercellular fluids, the quality of lymphatic fluids, and the quality of organs, tissues, and cells as well as their functions. Daily food largely shapes and determines our destiny in life. It is the major factor determining whether our natural immunity to infectious disease remains strong or weakens and decays.

Research has found that beneficial bacteria in the intestines synthesize many nutrients, including vitamins B and K, and strongly influence the internal balance of cholesterol and biliary compounds and acids and digestive juices which they produce. "It is important that the intestinal bacteria be properly fed (and not overfed)," explains Miles Robinson, M.D. "because a new generation occurs about every four hours, and it is characteristic of all bacteria to develop unsuitable and even virulent strains depending on how they are fed." Harmful strains are easily produced by consuming too much fat and dairy, too much sugar and highly processed foods, and not enough fiber. Such diets can produce diverticulitis, colon infections, digestive and circulatory diseases, diabetes, obesity, appendicitis, and gall bladder infections, as well as suppress immune function and set the stage for viral or bacterial infection.

Nearly all infectious diseases have been traced back to animals. Smallpox is derived from cowpox, influenza from avian or swine flu, and AIDS is associated with a simian immunodeficiency disease. Tuberculosis—a disease of cattle—often arises from excessive consumption of milk and other dairy food, and cholera is associated with chicken and eggs. In addition to physical proximity and shared living conditions and reliance on animal food, humans have also depended upon animals for fat for cooking, fur for clothing, and bones and sinews for tools. As Frank Fenner notes in an article in *Emerging Viruses*, conditions that facilitate human infection include viral epidemics "in wild animals in the agricultural areas and forest surrounding human settlements, the use of meat of wild animals as an important source of animal protein, and close contact of humans with wild animals, including such activities as trapping, killing, skinning, playing with carcases, and the consumption of raw or partially cooked meat."

Unlike plant-quality food, animal food begins to decompose immediately after it is slaughtered and to be consumed by a variety of microbes. By the time it reaches the intestines, animal food often contains microorganisms that can cause sickness, especially if the animal food is spoiled or in an advanced state of putrefaction. Even today, in a modern world of universal refrigeration and rigorous meat inspection, there are periodic outbreaks of food poisoning traced to tainted meat, eggs, poultry, or dairy.

4

Diet and Immune Deficiency

To understand the dietary cause of natural immune deficiency, it is convenient to classify food and modern eating habits into two general groupings:

• **The Yin Category:** Foods that produce a result or tendency toward expansion, decomposition, softening, loosening, and other similar effects of the muscles, tissues, organs, glands, and their functions.
• **The Yang Category:** Foods that produce a result or tendency toward contraction, composition, hardening, gathering, and other similar effects of the muscles, tissues, organs, glands, and their functions.

In a temperate climate, foods may be classified as follows:

Extreme Yang Foods

Refined salt	Poultry
Eggs	Fish
Meat	Seafood
Salty cheese	

Balanced Yin/Yang Foods

Whole-cereal grains
Beans and bean products
Sea vegetables
Root, round, and leafy
  vegetables

Whole seeds and nuts
Spring or well water
Nonaromatic, nonstimulant
  teas
Natural sea salt

Extreme Yin Foods

Temperate climate fruit
White rice, white flour
Tropical fruits and
  vegetables
Milk, cream, yogurt
Oils
Spices and herbs
Coffee, tea, and stimulants

Honey, sugar, and refined
  sweeteners
Alcohol
Foods containing chemi-
  cals, preservatives, dyes,
  pesticides
Drugs (marijuana, cocaine,
  etc.)

All foods are composed of both yin and yang characteristics but in different proportions. This categorization is a general rather than an absolute one, and varies depending upon the environment. In the modern way of eating, foods producing extreme yin or yang tendencies are customarily served or prepared together. Though they make a rough balance, they are often too extreme for daily eating. Examples include: meat and potatoes, meat and black pepper and other spices, turkey and cranberry sauce with herbs and gravy, lamb and mint jelly, clams and horseradish, hamburger and catsup and raw onions, hotdog and mustard, fish and lemon and oil, lobster and escargot and butter and garlic, cheese and tomatoes, cheese and wine, bacon and eggs with orange juice.

In general, overconsumption of animal food attracts sweets, stimulants, spices, oils, soft drinks, fruit and fruit juices, as well as nightshade plants such as potato, tomato, eggplant, and green and red peppers. Similarly, baked flour products attract sweets, oily spreads, and aromatic beverages, as well as more liquid including milk and beer.

These attempts to harmonize extremes often cannot achieve comprehensive balance and harmony in the long run and inevitably lead to disease and disorder at many levels. On the other hand, a macrobiotic way of eating based on a traditional diet centered around whole cereal grains and vegetables, supplemented with beans and legumes, fresh vegetables prepared in various ways, sea vegetables, and occasional consumption of fish and seafood, seasonal fruits, seeds and nuts, as well as nonstimulant beverages, can easily achieve more comprehensive harmony of nutrients, energies, and other factors contributing to physical health, mental well-being, and spiritual development.

Food can further be categorized into two groups of acid-producing roods and alkaline-producing foods. Examples include:

• **Acid-Producing Food:** Food containing more simple sugars, protein, and fat; food containing less fiber and minerals in general; food containing more water-soluble vitamins
• **Alkaline-Producing Food:** Food containing more complex sugars, less protein and fat; food containing more fiber and minerals in general; food containing more fat-soluble vitamins

A daily diet composed of rich animal meat, dairy food, sugar, fruits, refined products, and oily, greasy food, together with frequent consumption of tropical fruits, soft drinks, and aromatic, stimulant beverages—in other words, the modern way of eating—produces a more acidic condition within the body. On the other hand, traditional dietary practice consisting of whole unrefined grains, cooked vegetables, beans and their products, sea vegetables, and other natural foods seasoned with sea salt-based condiments and accompanied by nonstimulant beverages tend to produce a more alkaline condition in the body.

New diseases are emerging because of a change in food quality. For example, chocolate today is very different than chocolate twenty, thirty, or fifty years ago. New pesticides, preservatives, and other chemicals have been introduced.

New processing techniques have been developed. Greater amounts of carbon dioxide and pollutants have been released into the atmosphere. The end result is weaker blood and lymph, the emergence of new diseases, and the return of old ones that are resistant to drugs and vaccines.

Diet and Organ Weakness

According to our careful observation since the beginning of the current viral and bacterial epidemics, people who have weakened their natural immunity and are susceptible to infection share the same general dietary tendencies. These tendencies are:

• Consuming a great amount of sweets, including food containing sugar, chocolate, carob, honey, and chemical sweeteners.
• Consuming a great amount of fruits and fruit juices, including such tropical fruits as banana, papaya, mango, avocado, kiwi fruit, and others.
• Consuming a great amount of dairy products, especially milk, yogurt, cream, butter, ice cream, and food products containing them.
• Consuming refined flour products, including refined white flour, yeasted bread, and other baked products.
• Frequent consumption of nightshade plants such as tomato, potato, eggplant, and peppers, as well as plants that originated in a tropical climate.
• Consuming a great deal of oily and fatty food products, including salad dressing, spreads, sauces, and deep-fried foods.
• Frequent consumption of soft drinks and sparkling carbonated waters.

The items in these seven categories fall primarily within the category of extreme yin foods and beverages. They produce expanding, decomposing, loosening, and weakening results in various organs and glands and their functions. At the same time, these foods generate overwhelming acid-producing conditions in the body.

Because of the chronic consumption of these foods in excessive amounts, the following physical disorders arise:

1. Intestinal Weakness. The intestinal tract tends to become expanded and loose. Stagnation of bowel movements and sometimes constipation, but often diarrhea, and gas formation occur. Associated symptoms, such as colitis, may also appear, causing discomfort and suffering. Further, the activity of microorganisms in the intestines becomes chaotic, and their natural synthesizing function of necessary nutrients, including the important vitamin-B group, becomes deficient. A lack of the vitamin-B group further creates various disorders in body functions, including loss of clear judgment.

Further, weakened intestines cannot absorb food molecules effectively through the villi. This results in the deterioration of blood components including lymphocytes and other elements of the immune system. In addition, these extreme foods make the condition of the inside of the intestines abnormally acidic and leads to the formation of excess mucus and fatty acid. Parasites and other undesirable microorganisms including harmful viruses and bacteria thrive in this weakened internal environment and multiply rapidly.

2. Liver Infection, Hepatitis, and Mononucleosis. At some point, with or without conscious awareness, a liver infection occurs, often accompanied by fever. Chronic weakness of the liver and its various functions often continues for a long period despite medical treatment. When the liver is impaired, its primary function of storing excess nourishment in the form of glycogen and supplying stored nourishment to the bloodstream when required cannot work well. As a result, overeating becomes more frequent. Foods rich in sweets and easily digested foods are especially craved.

3. Lymphatic Disorder. In coordination with intestinal disorders and weakened liver function, the function of the spleen and its related lymphatic network tends to become chaotic. Spleen functions become weak, and the organ tends to enlarge. Lymph nodes also become swollen, and their func-

54

tion of cleansing poisonous waste from the lymphatic stream remains impaired. Because of the lack of minerals resulting from excessive consumption of the above mentioned food-stuffs, malfunction of the lymphatic system occurs. The symptoms of lymphoma—a cancerous condition of the lymphatic system—are often produced as a result.

4. **Weakening of Respiratory Function.** Weakening of the respiratory function results from the excessive consumption of foods in the extreme yin category and acid-forming foods. Sound respiratory functions become hindered. These foods also produce mucus, and fatty acid also gathers in the lungs. Symptoms of pneumonia or similar feverish disorders tend to occur occasionally or chronically. Breathing difficulties with accompanying fever are also often present.

Weakening of respiratory function interferes with the smooth supply of oxygen (O_2) to the red-blood cells and the proper elimination of carbon dioxide (CO_2). Disorders in blood components, including red-blood cells, white-blood cells, blood platelets, and blood plasma can result from respiratory disorder or from impairment of the intestinal, liver, and lymphatic functions. In any case, the condition of the blood and intercellular fluids worsens.

5. **Pancreatic Disorders.** One of the primary reasons for craving sweets, fruits, and other soothing foods in excessive amounts is due to chronic pancreatic disorder. The pancreas secretes two hormones, insulin and anti-insulin. Impairment in insulin secretion can lead to diabetes, while impairment in anti-insulin can lead to hypoglycemia, or chronic low blood sugar. Hypoglycemia results in frequent cravings for simple sugars or food rich in simple sugar including fruit and alcohol, as well as food rich in fatty acid. This condition of the pancreas is caused by excessive consumption of dairy fats, including cheese, as well as frequent consumption of poultry and eggs. In modern society, especially in the Western world, the consumption of these foods begins in early childhood and continues in adulthood, The fat from these foods is gathered in the pancreas and hinders the secretion of anti-insulin, which works to elevate the level of blood sugar. This results in a craving for simple sugar and wild, erratic changes in

emotions when the body's blood sugar levels drop, especially in the afternoon and evening. The majority of adults in modern Western society suffer from hypoglycemia to a varying degree.

6. Weakness of Bones. Because of the excessive consumption of acid-producing foods, including simple sugar, the pH factor of the blood tends to become more acidic, producing a tendency toward acidosis. To prevent this dangerous condition, the body's mineral reserves (especially stored calcium in the bones) are mobilized, to maintain a weak alkaline condition in the blood stream.

This buffer-action changes strong acid to weak acid and then further breaks it down to water (H_2O) and carbon dioxide (CO_2). The minerals required for this buffer action must be supplied in a daily diet that includes land and sea vegetables and other traditional foods high in vitamins and minerals, as well as moderate use of good-quality traditional, unrefined sea salt. Otherwise, the body will draw upon reserves in the bones, which results in a gradual weakening of the skeletal frame and degenerative conditions such as osteoporosis.

7. Skin Disorders. Because of the excessive consumption of simple sugar and fatty acid, body metabolism cannot support the active elimination of this dietary excess in most cases. Accordingly, the surface of the face and body becomes more milky in color with a red-pinkish shade. The milky texture is due to excessive consumption of dairy food, as well as oily, greasy food. Red-pinkish shades are due to expansion of the blood capillaries beneath the surface of the skin, resulting from overconsumption of foods in the extreme yin category, especially sweets, fruits, and others. In some cases, however, elimination of excessive dairy fats may appear on the skin in the form of white-yellowish patches. In other cases, the surface skin may not show these discolorations because fat layers are formed immediately below the skin which prevent elimination at the surface.

8. Skin Cancer—Kaposi's Sarcoma. In some cases of AIDS, the elimination of excess fat and protein, combined with excessive simple sugar, especially refined cane sugar, chocolate, honey, and others, results in a form of skin cancer.

As in the case of malignant melanoma, which is caused chiefly by excessive fat mainly from poultry, eggs, and cheese, and the case of skin cancer, mainly caused by excessive oily, greasy food, Kaposi's sarcoma is formed as a process of elimination toward the surface of the body by an undesirable combination of fat, protein and simple sugar. In many cases, excessive animal-quality protein may combine with these substances.

Kaposi's sarcoma appears in the form of dark, brownish-black marks and may spread all over the skin. They continuously appear and spread as long as excessive fat, protein and simple sugar remain within the system beyond the capacity of normal eliminatory functions, especially respiratory and urinary elimination. Kaposi's sarcoma can also appear in the inner lining of the oral cavity and gums, as well as inside the respiratory tract, the digestive tract, rectum, and anal region.

9. Reproductive Organ Disorder. Because of overconsumption of foods in the extreme yin category and of acid-producing foods, fatty acid and mucus gather in the reproductive organs such as the prostate and testes and the uterus and ovaries. In males, the condition may appear as a skin rash, as a red and white skin discoloring, and sensitivity at the time of urination. Other abnormal conditions may also appear. In females, this condition may manifest in a similar way and also in the form of vaginal discharge and vaginal and other localized infections.

The internal fluid in these regions becomes more acidic with various acid chemical compounds, including fatty acid, uric acid, sulphur compounds, and others. This condition creates a state easily receptive to viral growth and supports their activities. The degree of susceptibility to infectious viruses and bacteria such as those associated with gonorrhea, syphilis, herpes, and AIDS differs according to the strength of the individual's natural immunity and dietary habits.

10. Nervous Sensitivity. Because of the excessive consumption of foods from the extreme yin category, the peripheral nerves become more expanded and sensitized. Physical and chemical sensations and stimuli tend to produce overreactions. It becomes difficult to tolerate cold weather or withstand strong physical pressure or stress. Moving to a warmer climate in the winter, avoiding hard physical labor, and seeking relations only with similar types of people are typical lifestyle changes associated with this condition.

On the other hand, this tendency also sensitizes the nervous system, often creating a liking for delicate matters. Aesthetic appreciation of the arts and culture is often highly developed, producing a preference for certain types of occupations such as designing, furnishing, decorating, art work, music, hairdressing, and others activities that require more refined aesthetic sensitivity.

11. Mental Indecision. Overconsumption of foods in the extreme yin category and acid-producing foods gradually leads to the development of general indecisiveness, lack of clarity, and self-indulgence. Daily life tends to lack clear direction, and the person's ability to persevere in the face of difficulty and the ordinary vicissitudes of daily life declines.

Procrastination, timidity, and cowardice often develop, interfering with the person's overall direction in life and weakening their ambition, dream, and vision. Tenderness and kindness in human relations are demonstrated, and yet there is a general tendency for a lack of clear decision, resolution, and order.

A subconscious tendency to depend upon other people and circumstances arises. This mental tendency often results in a chaotic lifestyle lacking self-discipline, responsibility, and direction, as well as individual isolation or withdrawal into an exclusive group with those who share similar tendencies. This may manifest in feelings of religious, spiritual, moral, or aesthetic superiority and feelings that the body, physical health, and daily life on this planet are unimportant.

By improving eating habits in a more healthy direction, this mental tendency gradually changes toward more self-discipline, responsibility, ambition, and a positive and creative spirit and lifestyle.

12. Receptivity toward Infectious Viruses and Bacteria. In people who share the above physical and mental tendencies and lifestyles, infectious viruses and bacteria can be easily transmitted and multiply within the body. These microorganisms thrive in more acid-producing environments where excessive fat and mucus have accumulated, such as in the reproductive organs, the intestinal tract, and even the mouth cavity if an acidic condition arises. When these parts of the body make direct contact with an infected person or fluid carrying viruses and bacteria, the microorganism can be easily transmitted and may spread quickly.

If a dietary change takes place toward healthier eating practices, this receptivity to infectious viruses and bacteria would gradually decrease. As an overly acidic condition of fat and mucus is reduced, a more normal condition develops, and natural immunity may gradually be restored.

Natural immune deficiency develops in accordance with the physical and mental disorders and changes in lifestyle outlined above. These conditions develop gradually over a period of many years. The modern way of eating is a primary cause of natural immune deficiency. Dietary influence is not limited to childhood and adulthood. In some cases weakened natural immunity has already begun to develop during the period of pregnancy. During the embryonic period, energy and nutrients that support the formation of the body and associated functions are supplied through the placenta and the embryonic cord. If the mother's eating habits consisted largely of foods from the extreme yin category and acid-producing foods—including excessive consumption of animal protein and fat, dairy foods, simple sugars, fruits and fruit juices, soft drinks, chemicalized food and beverages, and others—a baby developing in the mother's womb may be born with a tendency toward natural immune deficiency. This orientation may manifest in symptoms of AIDS, especially if improper foods continue to be consumed after birth throughout the growing period, or susceptibility to infectious disease in general.

5

Lifestyle Factors

In addition to improper diet, many aspects of modern life promote and encourage the development of natural immune deficiency. Modern living is oriented toward satisfying sensory pleasure and emotional comfort through material prosperity. It largely sacrifices physical health, mental strength, and spiritual development. The problems of modern living are often treated symptomatically through technical applications emphasizing speed, convenience, and efficiency, ignoring a more comprehensive view that takes into account humanity's biological and spiritual nature. Various aspects of modern lifestyles and technology produce harmful effects that imperil the existence and continued development of humanity on this planet.

Some of the harmful aspects of modern life that promote natural immune deficiency can be outlined as follows:

1. Biological Orientation in the Embryonic Period. During pregnancy, from the time of conception to the time of birth, the human embryo increases in weight approximately 3 billion times. Formation of systems, organs, glands, and their related functions establish the human physical and mental constitution. Primary orientation for this development is made by hereditary genes such as DNA, but the quality and capacities of the human constitution are primarily developed through the energy and nutrients received through the placenta. The mother's eating habits largely shape and determine her baby's destiny. If the mother's way of eating is imbalanced, deformities may be produced including harelips, missing fingers or toes, multiple or transposed organs, retardation, and other abnormalities. At the same time, the quality and functional ability of systems, organs, and glands is also influenced.

In addition to dietary influence, parental consciousness—especially that of the mother—strongly influences the subconscious mind of the child. A mother with a calm, peaceful mind tends to produce a child with a peaceful orientation, while a mother with a disorderly, chaotic mind passes that attitude to the subconscious of her child.

The modern way of life tends to produce a child that is physically and mentally weaker than children were in the past. The size and weight of children today tend to be larger and heavier than necessary. Physical and mental response tends to be duller.

On the average, natural immunity is stronger in a smaller, thinner, and shorter child and weaker in a larger, fatter, and taller child. Compared with children from a few generations ago, modern children are weaker in their physical and mental resistance, endurance, and response in general. This means that modern newborns are also weaker in natural immunity than a few generations ago. This weakness prevails especially among children who were born after about 1950. At that time, dietary habits began to change dramatically with the use of chemicals in the production and processing of food, and food itself became more highly refined.

Following several years of social and economic reconstruction after World War II, the modern diet, including large amounts of meat, poultry, eggs, dairy food, and other animal products, along with sugar, soft drinks, canned and frozen food, white bread and white flour, and other highly processed foods, began to spread throughout society. At the same time, the trend toward economic depression and material sacrifice that preceded and followed the Second World War was followed in the 1950s and early 1960s by a conscious quest for physical comfort, sensory gratification, and mental pleasure.

2. Weakening of Natural Immunity at Birth. Because increasing numbers of newborns are physically larger and heavier and many mothers have weak contracting power during delivery, Caesarean surgery has tripled in modern society, accounting for about one in every five births. In addition, the use of forceps, drugs, and other emergency measures to assist in delivery has become more widespread.

If the newborn does not experience passing through the natural birth canal with strong repeated contractions, the child tends to be weaker in physical endurance and resistance in general.

At the same time, nursing is often intentionally stopped, and artificially produced formula is substituted for mother's milk. During the first few days after delivery, the mother's breast secretes a yellow fluid, called colostrum, which has ample immune factors. Throughout the next period of breast-feeding, as regular mother's milk is produced, the newborn continues to receive essential natural immune factors. These include antibodies that resist the growth of undesirable viruses and bacteria, provide immunity against infectious disease (especially rickettsia, salmonella, polio, influenza, strep, and staph), promote strong white-blood cells, and produce *B. bifidum*, a unique type of healthy bacteria found in the intestines of babies that creates resistance to a large variety of potentially harmful microorganisms. In a survey of sixty men with AIDS, Dr. Martha Cottrell found that all had been formula-fed with the exception of one who was breast-fed for less than three months.

These immune factors decrease as time passes. It is more difficult for the newborn to develop natural immunity if it has not been breastfed. Further, during these first few days, the newborn loses weight, contracting itself in order to acquire strength for adaption to the new environment.

The period of breastfeeding is very important in strengthening natural immunity. Upon birth, the newborn's living environment changes from the world of water in the uterus to the world of air on land. Naturally, the newborn is exposed to many kinds of new influences in the surrounding environment, including solar and celestial radiation, cosmic rays, and other influences of the universe, as well as the movement, pressure, temperature, and humidity of the atmosphere and many physical, chemical, and vibrational factors. Therefore, it is important for the newborn to develop natural immunity as smoothly as possible as a means of adapting to the environment and to resist undesirable factors including harmful viruses, bacteria, and other microorganisms as well as physical and chemical invasion and other adverse stimuli.

All mammal species depend upon breastfeeding directly from their mother. Breastfeeding supplies not only energy and nutrients but also confers immunity. If breastfeeding is replaced with artificial formulas which are produced for chemical and nutritional composition without careful consideration of natural immunity, the newborn may appear to grow satisfactorily, but it tends to be weaker, and its ability to adapt to its changing environment is diminished. Such a child may experience such undesirable symptoms as frequent colds, indigestion, diarrhea, skin rashes, allergies, complaining, oversensitivity, and other problems. Breast-fed infants, for example, have about one-fourth the risk of developing serious respiratory and gastrointestinal illnesses as bottle-fed infants, and one-tenth the risk of acquiring a life-threatening bacterial infection.

Though breastfeeding is desirable, circumstances may not always allow the mother to nurse her child. In such cases, food for the newborn should be carefully considered, including the quality and proportion of carbohydrate, protein, fats, vitamins, enzymes, and especially minerals. Until a few generations ago, it was common practice for newborns to be breastfed by other mothers as substitutes when a mother could not nurse the child herself.

In economically undeveloped societies, newborns who could not develop natural immunity sufficient for adapting to the new environment after birth would, in many cases, not survive to the age of three years. In modern society, health care, including improved sanitation, protects the newborn even when it does not develop sufficient immunity. However, this only postpones the problem to a future date. The child with weak immunity may well continue to survive if he or she is well-protected from the natural environment, like a plant growing in a hot house. Or if properly nourished, the child can develop natural immunity during the growing period.

3. Weakening of Natural Immunity During the Growing Period. In modern society, every individual faces many influences and occasions which weaken natural immunity. These include:

A. Change of Dietary Habits. Modern dietary habits have drastically changed, especially since the 1950s when a high-protein and high-fat diet became standardized in the United States and most of the industrialized world. Chemical agriculture replaced organic farming, and grain and flour products were increasingly refined. Commercially prepared fast food replaced home cooking, and modern advertising elevated sensory appeal and satisfaction, along with packaging, over such basic concerns as food quality and wholesomeness. This vast, fundamental change in the modern way of eating has naturally altered the biological, mental, and spiritual status of human beings, contributing to degenerative disease and the weakening of natural immunity. The lack of whole grains and natural minerals in fresh vegetables has particularly contributed to the decline of natural immune functions.

The cooking methods favored by modern food technology—electricity and microwave—have also changed food quality. Cooking by wood, charcoal, gas, and other natural fuels maintains the harmonious unity of foods, while electricity, microwave, and other highly refined forms of heating tend to decompose food molecules, creating chaotic energy and a disorderly vibration. Stanford medical researchers reported that microwaving breast milk destroyed 98 percent of its immunolobulin-A antibodies and 96 percent of its liposome activity that inhibits bacterial growth. German scientists reported that microwave cooking reduced hemoglobin and lymphocyte levels and raised leukocyte counts and levels of light-emitting bacteria. They concluded that the subjects were

64

responding to the food as if it were an infectious agent. Microwave cooking has now spread from many public establishments to private homes. About 80 percent of all American families report having a microwave oven, and a majority use them regularly. Teflon and other chemically-treated types of nonstick cookware have also spread. In the United States today, 75 percent of the pots and pans sold are coated with synthetic materials. Growing up, every person today is exposed more or less to this type of food and cooking, and their natural immunity may be weakened as a result.

B. Abuse of Medication. In modern daily life, the use of drugs and pills is nearly universal. Sleeping pills, digestive pills and aids, aspirin and pain killers, tranquilizers and sedatives, and other medications and drugs are widely used as a normal part of daily life in the majority of families. The use of over-the-counter and prescription drugs and pills has constantly grown over the past several decades. However, many of them produce a very acidic condition in the body, which directly contributes to the weakening of natural immunity.

C. Removal of Tonsils and Other Glands. The majority of adults in modern society have had their tonsils and adenoids surgically removed during childhood to prevent tonsilitis. However, this is based on a deep misunderstanding of the nature and function of these glands. Tonsillitis (inflammation of the tonsils) does not occur because of the existence of the tonsils. It occurs because of excessive consumption of food rich in simple sugars and fat. The tonsils are one of several important immune glands that serve to cleanse toxins, excess mucus, and other substances from the lymph system. Chronic swelling and inflammation show that they are doing their job of localizing and neutralizing dietary excess. The way to relieve tonsilitis is not to take out the tonsils but to stop the intake of improper foods and drinks that are overburdening the lymphatic system. If the tonsils are removed, infectious diseases can spread more easily.

D. Exposure to X-Rays. Unlike our ancestors, the overwhelming majority of people in modern society have been exposed to X-rays on various occasions such as during medical and dental examinations. Frequent exposure to X-rays may increase the risk of certain kinds of cancer, including leukemia and lymphoma. It also weakens natural immunity.

E. Exposure to Other Radiation. In modern life, daily exposure to artificial electromagnetic radiation is often experienced, including that from television, computers, cellular phones, and other electronic equipment. Furthermore, throughout the atmosphere and underground, some regions of the earth have been exposed to large amounts of undesirable radiation caused by the use of nuclear energy and nuclear explosions. Because radiation—both ionizing and non-ionizing, though to differing degrees—gives yin, expansive, decomposing, and in some cases freezing effects, it contributes to the decline of natural immunity. Irradiation of food may also produce similar effects over an extended period of time. Further, the loss of ozone in the earth's atmosphere has increased humanity's exposure to potentially dangerous ultraviolet radiation. Ultraviolet damage to the surface of the skin weakens natural immunity and may result in the increase of infectious diseases. Ozone loss is caused primarily from chloroflurocarbons (CFC) used in aerosol sprays, plastics, computers and electronics, and other industrial applications.

F. Drug Abuse. The use of drugs has soared since the 1960s, especially among older adolescents and young adults. These include marijuana, mescaline, LSD, and other hallucinogenic substances; amphetamines and barbituates; and heroin, cocaine, and other narcotics. These drugs give more yin, expanding and decomposing effects to physical and mental conditions and have the effect of dulling the functions of the nervous system. The overall result contributes to the weakening of natural immune functions.

G. Abuse of Medical Treatment. In modern society, medical treatment has become the standard method of treating sickness. Because degenerative disease is so prevalent and modern people experience so much physical and mental decline, medical treatment has sometimes been overused. Removal of the appendix without the actual occurrence of appendicitis causes unnecessary weakening of the intestinal functions in many cases. Similarly, the excessive use of medication and surgical operations causes the decline of natural immunity. Chemotherapy and other strong drug applications, although they may be required in some cases, tend to weaken natural immunity by changing the quality of the blood, including decreasing the number of white-blood cells. Mercury amalgam fillings in teeth may leech into the mouth and bloodstream, weakening the body.

H. Overuse of Antibiotics. Antibiotics have been employed successfully for the past several decades to deal with bacterial infections. However, the use of antibiotics tends to change and weaken the activities of beneficial microorganisms in the digestive system, especially in the intestines. This causes disorders in the digestive functions and contributes to the decline of natural immunity. In general, the use of drugs to weaken or suppress viral and bacterial activities may also cause the deterioration of normal healthy microorganisms which, in turn, further contribute to the decline of natural immunity. Moreover, in recent years, new strains of microorganisms have developed that are resistant to ordinary doses of antibiotics. They require ever-stronger drugs to control, further weakening natural immunity.

I. Environmental Pollution. Despite more public awareness of industrial and chemical pollution, much of the planet's land, water, and air has been polluted. Acid rain damages crops, forests, and biological life in rivers and lakes. Nuclear wastes and radioactive substances are contaminating the atmosphere, water, and ground, endangering life at all levels. Chemicals and toxic wastes dumped into lakes, rivers, and oceans are destroying marine life, while pesticides and other chemical sprays used on fields and forests are killing wild animals and birds.

In metropolitan areas, pollution from automobiles, airplanes, and industry is also poisoning the atmosphere. Abnormal electromagnetic influences from power plants, high-voltage power lines, and communication facilities are also damaging human health and the environment. Apart from pollution in the external environment, overly insulated modern houses often pollute interior environments through use of synthetic building materials and other artificially treated substances, and air-conditioning can spread potentially harmful microbes.

As a result of worldwide environmental pollution, all animal life, including human life, is under threat of deformation, weakening, degeneration, and even possible extinction.

J. Promiscuous Sexual Behavior. Due to the weakened natural immunity of modern people, viral and bacterial infections can be easily spread, especially among those whose lifestyle includes promiscuous sexual behavior. Since the sexual revolution of the 1960s, the incidence of sexually transmitted diseases (STD), including herpes and others, has risen dramatically.

From early childhood, most young people today have been exposed to sexually explicit material in books, magazines, on television, in films, and in the home, school, and community. As society's attitude toward sexual behavior has become more permissive, many of them have begun to have sexual encounters at an earlier age. As a result, there is a tendency among modern people to select sexual partners carelessly. Together with decline of spiritual intuition and biological instinct, the ability to choose an appropriate partner has declined, and promiscuous sexual behavior has increased. Compared to the recent past, the potential number of carriers of infectious viruses and bacteria has soared.

In the case of heterosexuals, physical contact with prostitutes is one of the major potential sources of infection. In the case of homosexuals, sexual activity is often accompanied by drug use. Also, among various forms of sexual intercourse, oral and anal intercourse have a higher risk of lowering natural immunity than vaginal intercourse, because semen contains acid-forming compounds, along with sulphur, ammonia, and uric acid, in addition to simple fatty acids, which contribute to an overall acidic internal environment. In the case of seminal fluid, the yin decomposing power of sperm and male reproductive follicles is roughly one hundred times greater than simple sugar or other extreme dietary yin. Frequent anal or oral sex, in which semen is absorbed into the blood and lymphatic stream through the digestive system, would have the overall effect of lowering natural immunity.

6

Environmental and Social Factors

As we have seen, viral and bacterial infection and communication are activated by more yin tendencies—expansion, decomposition, dilution. Loss of energy arising from these tendencies also stimulates microbial activities.

This view helps us understand the incidence and spread of AIDS and infectious disease in general. The sociological profile that emerges is as follows:

1. Microbial infections tend to arise and spread more in warmer climatic regions than in colder ones. Practically speaking, tropical and semitropical areas are affected more than northern areas and areas closer to the polar regions.

2. Microbes are more active in the summer and less active in the winter in temperate regions. For example, in central Europe or most parts of North America, we could expect a more rapid increase of viral and bacterial activity in late spring, summer, and early autumn and a slower increase in late autumn, winter, and early spring.

3. There is more microbal activity in a humid environment than a dry one. There is more activity in a rainy season than in a dry one.

4. There is more microbial activity in cities with large populations than in rural areas with smaller populations. Ur-

ban regions suffer more than villages and towns.

5. Microbial activity is greater where sanitary conditions are lacking.

6. Infection is more likely among social sectors that consume larger amounts of food rich in animal protein and fat, including dairy food; food rich in simple sugar such as refined cane sugar, chocolate, honey, ice cream, and soft drinks; and fruit and fruit juice, especially of a tropical and semitropical nature. Microbial activity is also be greater among people who consume large amounts of acid-producing food, including the above mentioned items, vegetables of the nightshade family, and oily, greasy food.

7. Infection is greater in communities that depend more heavily upon the transportation of food from a different climatic region, especially a hotter and more humid zone.

8. Infection is higher where drug abuse is prevalent and where promiscuous sexual activity is practiced.

9. In temperate regions, males are affected more frequently than females because they are more easily weakened by yin acid-producing food such as simple sugar, fruit, and alcohol. However, in hot tropical regions, both males and females are affected about equally.

10. There is a greater risk of microbial infection among the population born after 1950.

11. The risk of infection is greater among people engaged in sexual relationships with multiple partners rather than monogamous relationships.

12. Infections are more common among homosexual men than lesbian women because risk factors as noted above are more predominant among males than females.

From this pattern, it would be possible to draw a map projecting the future development and spread of AIDS and other infectious conditions. At the same time, this pattern would help epidemiologists and other scientific and medical researchers investigate possible counterbalancing dietary and environmental factors that could help prevent or slow epidemic trends in different regions of the world.

AIDS in the Tropics

Though AIDS is now global, affecting practically every culture and nation, it is spreading most rapidly in the tropical regions of the world, including Africa, Latin America, India and Pakistan, and other warmer latitudes. The unifying principle of yin and yang helps us understand the incidence and spread of AIDs. Viral infections, as well as infectious conditions caused by bacteria, parasites, and other organisms, spread more rapidly in warm, hot regions where people are balancing the yang contracted environment with proportionately more yin expansive food and beverages. In many tropical countries, people are no longer eating a diet centered around whole grains and vegetables like their ancestors. Instead, they are eating large amounts of sugar, spices, oil, stimulant beverages, nightshade plants, and other items with strong yin energy, as well as animal food, dairy food, refined flour, highly processed foods, and other foods imported from the West. Uprooted from their traditional farmland to make way for cattle ranching, sugar plantations, and other aspects of modern agriculture and food production, they have flocked to cities and urban slums where they are subject to malnutrition, unemployment, and destitution. Well meaning relief agencies then compound the problem by distributing evaporated milk and infant formula, canned goods, refined grains, sugar, and other high caloric items. HIV, as well as many other infectious organisms, breed in such an environment.

Several years ago, I was invited to give a seminar to medical doctors and World Health Organization officials in West Africa, where AIDS has reached epidemic proportions. I observed that AIDS was frequent in big cities and among people eating in the modern way, but in the rural areas where grains, vegetables, and other more natural foods were still eaten, AIDS was much less common.

Over the years, I have met many young men with AIDS or borderline AIDS who go to the Caribbean or other warm, tropical climate for vacation. There tropical fruits including bananas, mango, gauva, pineapple, and papaya are plentiful, along with rum and alcohol, marijuana and cocaine, and other extreme yin substances. For AIDS, these are suicide zones. In addition to the food quality, the hot weather allows the virus to spread more quickly. For recovering from AIDS, a colder, more temperate climate is advisable.

AIDS in Men and Women

Females get AIDS much less than males. The reason for this is that they are constitutionally better able to take in yin than men. Conversely, men can handle yang better. Traditionally, women ate proportionately more vegetables, especially salad, fruit, sweets, desserts, and other yin foods and beverages, while men ate more animal food, more salt, more baked food, and other more yang items. Females have a hard time with yang foods—salty, baked food, eggs, meat, chicken, fish, etc.—and their intake in modern society by women and girls tends to make them hard, aggressive, and irritable and underlies the spread of uterine and ovarian tumors, lung cancer, and other yang disorders. Conversely, men have a hard time handling strong yin, such as too much fruit, juice, salad, ice cream, dairy food, and sugar. These foods have a tendency to make them weak, tired, and passive and predispose them to leukemia, lymphoma, AIDS, and other yin disorders. Overall, women are healthier than men and live longer because they are able to exchange energy more harmoniously with the environment through menstruation and lactation. Breastfeeding contributes to the health of the mother, as well as the child, and strengthens her natural immunity to disease.

The Spread of Microbial Infection

In spite of possible production of microbes, including AIDS-related viruses, within the body, especially in the blood, body fluids, in the interior of the intestines, and within the reproductive organs, through degeneration of primitive cells, the transmission of microbes from one person to another is currently a major means of spreading AIDS and other infections.

Since each person has a different degree of natural immunity and receptivity to viruses, the current health or already existing degenerative condition of a person is the underlying factor that determines the susceptibility and degree of infection. Even if exposed to harmful microorganisms, the metabolism of a healthy body harmonizes or neutralizes the undesirable viruses and bacteria by naturally producing antibodies.

The possible means of transmitting infectious microorganisms are generally as follows:

1. Sexual Intercourse. In the event a partner carries HIV, it could be transmitted to another partner during sexual intercourse. Transmission is made more easily through blood and bodily fluids high in acid, fat, and mucus, and fluid that is rich in nitrogen, sulfur, and ammonium compounds, uric acid, methane gas and other gaseous states, and others. Accordingly, primary means of transmission include: a) vaginal intercourse, b) anal intercourse, and c) oral intercourse. In the case of oral intercourse, the risk of transmission is higher for the male receiver than the female receiver.

Although the act of kissing exchanges fluid, the possibility of transmitting the virus remains small. The strong yang alkaline condition of the saliva helps neutralize the yin acid nature of the viruses.

2. Physical Contact. Simple physical contact such as shaking hands, touching, hugging, and caressing will not transmit HIV. However, if the skin's surface has an open wound, ulcerated rupture, cancerous condition, or allergic rash, transmission may occur through these sites. Air-borne microbes such as that associated with tuberculosis and water-borne microbes such as that associated with cholera may be spread by simple contact.

3. Blood Transfusion. Microbes can also be transmitted through contaminated blood. A blood transfusion is frequently needed for those who have lost a substantial amount of blood by accident, injury, or any other reason including hemophilia, leukemia, or malnutrition. The blood used for a transfusion, in most cases, is blood collected from donors and stored in a blood bank. There is a possibility that some of this blood carries harmful microbes, especially that of donors who have abused drugs, engaged in promiscuous sexual activity, or practiced chaotic eating habits. The pathogens in stored blood can be eliminated by heat treatment, but this treatment may not have been applied in some cases. The safest measure of blood transfusion is to collect blood from a member of the immediate family, relative, or close friend who has the same blood type and whose blood has been tested for safety prior to the transfusion.

4. **Blood Supplements.** Consumption of blood in the health-care field has greatly increased over the past several decades. In addition to blood transfusions, blood is utilized in the form of various tablets taken to boost energy and restore vitality. These tablets are also used for hemophilia, leukemia, and in cases where there has been a loss of blood. Until 1984, no precautions were taken to test such forms of blood for AIDS-related viruses. Blood supplements in tablet form have been distributed by manufacturers and they have been consumed by great numbers of people primarily in modern industrial societies. Accordingly, users of such supplements may be at higher risk for AIDS-related conditions.

5. **Eating and Drinking.** If harmful microbes are present in the food and water supply, there is a possibility of their reaching our digestive system and bloodstream. Contaminated meat and dairy food has been linked to recent *salmonella* and *E. Coli* outbreaks. Some water in rural areas in hot climates, especially those with high humidity and stagnant conditions, can also spread disease. When we take these foods and water without proper processing—such as cooking at high temperature and adding salt or minerals—transmission could occur. On the other hand, chlorinated and other chemically treated water can kill beneficial microbes in our body, making us more susceptible to infection.

6. **The Use of Needles and Instruments.** The AIDS virus and other microbes may also be transmitted by contaminated hypodermic needles and other unsterilized medical instruments. Needles are often used to inject chemicals or nutrients

in the blood, lymphatic stream, and into the tissues. Needles are also used in acupuncture treatment and other therapies. Among drug users, the needles are often circulated among a group without proper sanitation or sterilization.

Furthermore, invasive instruments are often used in the cases of intravenous injections, surgery, dental treatment, abortion, chemotherapy, and others. Unless these instruments are properly sanitized prior to their use, there is a possible risk of infection through these means. Current medical studies indicate that on average about two-thirds of doctors and one-third of nurses do not wash their hands or follow other routine hygienic procedures in the modern hospital or clinical setting.

7. **Embryonic Transmission.** In the event that a mother carries AIDS-related viruses in her body fluids, though she may not have any apparent symptoms herself it is quite possible that her baby could be infected through the umbilical cord, as well as through the fluids directly contacting the fetus. As the AIDS epidemic spreads, there will be increasing numbers of newborn infants who already carry viruses at birth. This degenerative trend alone gravely threatens humanity's continued existence, especially toward the beginning of the next century when the logarithmic increase of this number begins to become apparent.

8. **Transmission by Insects.** In tropical regions, it is well documented that mosquitos can transmit malaria, yellow fever, and other diseases. There has been speculation that AIDS-related viruses may also be transmitted by insects. Medical researchers have found no evidence to date of transmission from this source. However, such transmission remains a theoretical possibility and may require further investigation. Even if transmission by insects does not occur, infection caused by insects may serve to lower natural immunity. Generally, mosquitoes are attracted to the blood of people eating sugar, fruit, and other sweet-tasting foods.

9. **Technological transmission.** Air-conditioning, airplane and cruise ship ventilation, and supermarket food misters have been associated with spreading Legionnaire's disease, pneumonia, flu, or other infectious conditions.

7

Symptoms and Diagnosis of Disease

After contracting AIDS-related viruses, the symptoms of infection start to show up in various ways and degrees. They may appear within two months or they may not appear for several years. At the same time, the nature and degree of the symptoms are different and varied.

These variations are due to the individual's lifestyle and dietary habits, as well as the degree to which a person might have lowered his or her natural immunity prior to contracting the virus. However, the common symptoms are generally as follows:

1. General Fatigue. Both mentally and physically, the individual gradually loses his or her vitality. Ambition, endurance, and ability to meet challenges, as well as positive and optimistic attitudes, all decline. As a result, the person grows more inactive and seeks more comfortable situations and surroundings.

2. Development of Colds and Infections. Because of natural immune deficiency, viral and bacterial infections can easily occur. Such individuals often suffer from colds and infections accompanied by light fevers.

3. Skin Rashes. Similar to allergic infections, red and white rashes appear in some cases on the skin. These result from the elimination of infectious material on the surface of the skin together with excessive fatty substances.

4. Intestinal Disorders. Such individuals often suffer from gas formation, constipation, and frequent diarrhea. In the case of diarrhea, parasites may also be involved.

5. Feeling of Nausea. Some individuals frequently experience the feeling of nausea. Usually it occurs after eating or drinking. However, actual vomiting does not often arise.

6. Irregular Appetite. Appetite is often disturbed. At times people with AIDS or related symptoms may have a great appetite for food, but at other times they may have almost no appetite. Furthermore, they may favor certain types of food such as sweets or fruits. Food preferences may also change frequently.

7. Night Perspiration. During sleep, especially at night between midnight and early morning, abnormal perspiration may occur in some cases. It may be associated with a light fever and shivering.

8. Chronic Hypoglycemia. The individuals usually experience symptoms associated with hypoglycemia, including a tendency to be more mentally depressed, irritable, and pessimistic, particularly in the afternoon. Feelings of exhaustion occur during the night even while sleeping. Peripheral parts of the body such as the hands and feet are colder than normal in temperature. Cravings for simple sugars are also strong.

9. Liver Infection. Weakness of liver functions often appears. It may take the chronic form of hepatitis, mononucleosis, and other similar infections.

10. Swelling of Lymph Glands. The lymph glands, especially in the groin, armpit, neck and chest area, often become swollen in order to cope with viral activity. These conditions may develop to lymphatic cancer—lymphoma.

11. Abnormal Balance of Blood Components. Within the bloodstream, the white-blood cells tend to continuously decrease, but lymphocytes in particular decrease markedly. The ratio of immunity-related cells such as T4 and T8 cells changes. The number of T4 cells progressively decreases, and the ratio between the two becomes less than 1.0 and may even reach 0.1 or lower, which is one of the indications of very low immunity.

12. Pneumocystis Carinii. Some individuals may develop pneumocystis carinii accompanied by a state of chronic fever in which the body temperature tends to rise more in the evening and night than in the daytime. A chronic low-temperature fever, however, may continue over several months. As the situation develops, difficulty in breathing may tend to arise.

13. Kaposi's Sarcoma. In about 15 percent of cases, individuals develop Kaposi's sarcoma, which is cancer appearing on the skin. In the beginning, it may appear as a simple dark spot of small size. Gradually the number of spots may cover various body surfaces. The sarcoma may also arise in the cavity of the mouth, especially in the upper region, and in some cases around the anus. These spots are dark black or brown in color and semi-soft in texture. They are the result of the active elimination of excessive protein, fat, and simple sugars on the surface of the body, though in some cases this may happen within the interior of the digestive vessel and the respiratory tract.

14. Tuberculosis. TB can arise in the bones and joints, kidneys, bladder, intestines, lymph glands, or in any part of the body, but the most common form develops in the lungs. In the primary stage, the lymph nodes in the central part of the lung, around the entrance to the bronchi, become enlarged and calcified as the body's mineral reserves are depleted to counterbalance the acidic condition arising from repeated consumption of extreme yin and yang food. In this stage, the disease is considered to be non-infectious. The secondary stage is characterized by the formation of cavities in the lungs which continue to calcify and increase in size, causing the inner lung tissue to decompose. At this stage, the disease is actively infectious, since the many bacteria which thrive in the highly acidic environment of the lung cavities are often transmitted through breathing.

There are many other symptoms which may appear in relation to AIDS-related viral infections. Strictly speaking, the symptoms are different according to the individual, but on

the average the ability to adapt to the environment and to resist undesirable conditions within the environment declines.
Ultimately, the condition will deteriorate to the point that basic life activity as a human being can no longer be sustained.

Diagnosis of Disease

Modern society diagnoses AIDS by blood tests which show
the presence of antibodies to the HIV in the body. However,
since people may not symptomatize for years, millions of
men and women are believed to be carrying the HIV virus
without knowing it. When symptoms appear, it is often too
late for them to begin to reverse it. From the modern medical
view, AIDS is considered incurable and the most that can be
done is to prolong life through experimental drugs and to
minimize pain and suffering. From the macrobiotic view,
AIDS or a tendency toward loss of natural immunity can be
evaluated through traditional Oriental physiognomic methods.

Visually, a person with AIDS or carrying the AIDS virus
appears to have little vitality or energy, the face is red or
purply (a color that may show an infectious condition), the
movement or action is slow, the texture of the skin is milky,
the skin easily ruptures, the intestines are loose and diarrhea
may arise frequently. About half of the AIDS cases I have
seen had hepatitis or other liver disorders. In another 20 to 30
percent, the spleen or lymph nodes are swollen and expanded
and lymphoma arises. Eighty percent or more have hypoglycemia, or chronically low blood-sugar, from long-time consumption of dairy products, poultry, eggs, and other fatty
foods which gather and harden the pancreas. Hormones cannot release properly, and to relax they constantly crave
sweets, fruits, and other strong yin. Pre-AIDS conditions, in
my experience, are mononucleosis, chronic fatigue syndrome,
and Epstein-Barr virus.

8

Recovery from Disease

According to modern medicine, becoming infected with HIV amounts to a death sentence. There is no cure. From the macrobiotic view, this is not necessarily true. First, the aim is to keep the virus dormant. If dormant, a person can live ten, twenty, thirty years or more in relatively good health, and there is no need to worry. For those newly infected, the standard macrobiotic diet will often keep the virus inactive and the person symptom-free. For cases that have already begun to symptomatize, it can take two to three years to become normal, and then five to seven years in total for the virus to disappear completely from the body. Of course, some cases of AIDS are so far advanced that recovery is not possible. But still, improvement in the quality of life, reduced need for medical treatment and hospitalization, and a quiet, peaceful death at home makes it worthwhile to observe this approach.

The Macrobiotic Research on AIDS

In 1983 a group of men in New York City with AIDS began macrobiotics under my auspices. They hoped to change their blood quality, recover their natural immunity, and prolong their life. In May, 1984 a research team led by Elinor N. Levy, Ph.D. and John C. Beldekas, Ph.D. of the Department of Immunology and Microbiology at Boston University's School of Medicine and Martha C. Cottrell, M.D., then Director of Student Health at the Fashion Institute of Technology in New

York, began to monitor the blood samples and immune functions of men with Kaposi's sarcoma (a usual symptom of AIDS). Preliminary results indicated that most of the men were stabilizing on the diet. "Survival in these men who have received little or no medical treatment appears to compare very favorably with that of KS patients in general," the researchers reported in a letter to the *Lancet*, the British medical journal, in July, 1985. "We suggest that physicians and scientists can feel comfortable in allowing patients, particularly those with minimal disease, to go untreated as part of a larger [dietary] study or because non-treatment is the patient's choice."

At the International AIDS Conference in Paris in June, 1986, the researchers presented further findings concerning the men in the macrobiotic study:

1. The lymphocyte number increased over the first two years from disagnosis with KS in men who were following a macrobiotic diet. A statistical model predicted that the lymphocyte number would become normal within a two-year period.

2. During this time period, the percentage of T4 cells did not change. The percentage of T8 cells possibly decreased.

3. These results compared favorably with those from any of the medical treatments reported.

4. There were several possible explanations for these positive findings including: a) the macrobiotic diet and/or lifestyle was of benefit and b) the decision to become and remain macrobiotic selected for men with a better prognosis.

In a further report, Dr. Levy noted in 1988: "The large majority of subjects reported a decrease in AIDS-related symptoms, particularly fatigue (23/29) and diarrhea (17/19). The lymphocyte number in the subgroup of nineteen subjects with Kaposi's sarcoma alone tended to increase with time after diagnosis. Only two of this group of nineteen lost more than 10 percent of their body weight during their participation in the study which ranged from several months to more than three years. Nine of the nineteen with KS have died, seven are alive more than three years after diagnosis with KS."

In a letter to the American Cancer Society, Dr. Cottrell added, "The approach has demonstrated effective in managing their condition while minimizing opportunistic infections and use of toxic drugs. They are all working full time and enjoying a quality of life atypical of most AIDS patients. Most of all, they are relatively free of the sense of hopelessness, helplessness, and victimization which tends to take hold of other AIDS patients. Thus the physical benefits—prolonging life and improving the immunocompetence—seems complemented by a range of psychological benefits."

For further information on these studies, including case histories of some of the men involved, please see *AIDS, Macrobiotics, and Natural Immunity* by Michio Kushi and Martha Cottrell, M.D. with Mark Mead (Japan Publications, 1990) and *The Way of Hope: Michio Kushi's Anti-AIDS Program* by Tom Monte (Warner Books, 1990).

Dietary Recommendations

The following daily dietary recommendations are for persons with AIDS, those who have tested positive for HIV, or anyone else who is at high risk for AIDS. They are also beneficial for other immune-deficiency or autoimmune disorders such as environmental illness (EI), systemic lupus erythematosus (SLE), Epstein-Barr virus (EBV), cytomegalovirus (CMV), and chronic fatigue syndrome (CFS). Please note that these are average guidelines and need to be modified for each individual. We highly recommend that an experienced macrobiotic teacher be consulted regarding personal dietary practice.

The primary cause of AIDS and other immune-deficiency diseases is longtime consumption of excessive yin foods and beverages, along with other extreme yin influences including drugs and medication, exposure to artificial electromagnetic fields, and other factors that lower natural immunity to disease. All sugar, chocolate, honey, sweets, spices, herbs, soft drinks, wine, alcohol, fruit, juice, coffee, chemicalized tea, and other stimulants, foods of tropical origin, and oily, greasy foods of all kinds must be avoided. Because they are excessively mucus-producing, all flour products are to be avoided except for occasional consumption of nonyeasted unleavened whole-wheat or rye bread if craved. Chemicalized and artificially produced and treated foods and beverages are to be completely eliminated. Even unsaturated vegetable oil is to be completely avoided or minimized in cooking for a one- or two-month period. All ice-cold foods and drinks should be avoided. While AIDS is caused by more yin conditions, it is important not to yangize too quickly. If you try to strengthen yourself by taking too much good quality yang, such as whole grains, sea salt, sea vegetables, etc. the opposite problems may arise, including tightness and rigidity. The idea is to make balance, reducing yin, with slightly more emphasis on yang.

• **Whole Grains:** Fifty to sixty percent of daily consumption, by volume, should be whole-cereal grains. The first day prepare plain pressure-cooked short-grain brown rice. Then alternate brown rice cooked with 20 to 30 percent millet, then rice with 20 to 30 percent barley, then rice with 20 to 30 percent aduki beans or lentils. A delicious morning porridge can be made by taking leftover rice, adding a little more water to make soft, and seasoning with a little miso at the end and simmering for 2 to 3 minutes more. Except for morning porridge, which may be soft, the grain should be cooked in a ratio of 2 parts grain to 1 part water. For seasoning, cook with a small postage stamp-sized piece of kombu instead of salt, though in some cases sea salt may be used depending on the person's condition. Other grains can be used occasionally including whole-wheat berries, rye, corn, and, after the first month, whole oats. Buckwheat and seitan (wheat gluten) should be minimized. Good quality sourdough bread may be enjoyed 2 to 3 times a week and noodles, both udon and soba, may also be taken. Avoid all hard baked products until the condition improves including cookies, cake, pie, crackers, muffins, and the like.

• **Soup:** Five to ten percent soup, consisting of one or two cups or bowls per day of soup cooked with wakame sea vegetable and various land vegetables such as onions and carrots and seasoned with miso or shoyu. Occasionally a small volume of shiitake mushroom may be added to the soup. The miso may be barley miso, brown rice miso, or soybean (hatcho) miso and should be naturally aged two to three years. To satisfy a desire for a sweet taste, millet soup with sweet vegetables such as squash, cabbage, onions, and carrots may be prepared often. Grains soups, bean soups, and other soups may be taken from time to time.

• **Vegetables:** Twenty to thirty percent vegetables, cooked in a variety of forms, with plenty of hard, green leafy vegetables which are good for the liver and detoxification, round vegetables such as squash, cabbage, and onions which are good for the spleen and immune system, and root vegetables such as daikon, carrot, and burdock which are strengthening to the intestines and the blood and lymph as a whole. As a rule of thumb, the following dishes may be prepared, though the frequency may differ from person to person: *nishime*-style (longtime stewed) vegetables 3 to 4 times a week; squash-aduki-kombu dish 3 times a week; dried daikon, one cup, 3 times a week; carrots and carrot tops or daikon and daikon tops, 3 times a week; boiled salad 5 to 7 times a week; pressed salad, 5 to 7 times a week; raw salad and salad dressing, avoid; steamed greens, 5 to 7 times a week; sautéed vegetables, use water the first month instead of oil, then occasionally a small volume of sesame oil may be brushed on the skillet; *kinpira*-style (matchsticks), sautéed in water, two-thirds of a cup, 2 times a week, then oil may be used after three weeks; dried tofu, tofu, temphe, or seitan with vegetables, 2 times a week. As a special dish, vegetable *nabe* (lightly boiled vegetables and noodles cooked homestyle on the table) may be eaten frequently.

• **Beans:** Five percent small beans, such as azuki beans, lentils, chickpeas, or black soybeans, may be used daily, cooked together with sea vegetables such as kombu or with onions and carrots. Other beans may be used altogether 2 to 3 times a month. For seasoning, a small volume of unrefined sea salt or shoyu or miso can be used. Bean products, such as tempeh, natto, and dried or cooked tofu may be used occasionally but in moderate volume. Avoid making the tofu too creamy and use firm rather than soft tofu.

• **Sea Vegetables:** Five percent or less sea vegetable dishes, including wakame and kombu daily when cooking grain, in soup, etc. A sheet of toasted nori may also be taken daily. A small dish of hijiki or arame should be prepared two times a week. All other sea vegetables are optional.

• **Condiments:** Condiments to be available on the table are gomashio (sesame salt), on the average made with 1 part salt to 18 parts sesame seeds (reduced to 1:16 after 2 months), kombu, kelp, or wakame powder, umeboshi plum, and tekka, though all other regular macrobiotic condiments may be used if desired. These condiments may be used daily on grains and vegetables, but the volume should be moderate to suit individual appetite and taste. Umeboshi (1/2 to 1 plum a day) and tekka (1/4 to 1/3 teaspoon a day) are good for restoring immune ability.

• **Pickles:** Pickles, made at home in a variety of ways, are to be eaten daily, 1 teaspoon in all, though long-time salty pickles are to be minimized.

• **Animal Food:** Though animal food is to be avoided, a small volume of white-meat fish may be eaten once every week or two weeks. The fish should be prepared steamed, boiled, or pouched and be garnished with grated daikon or ginger. After two months, fish may be eaten once or twice a week and may be prepared with other cooking styles such as broiling, grilling, and baking. Strictly avoid blue-meat and red-meat fish and all shellfish. For energy and vitality, *koi koku* (carp soup) may be taken if desired, 1 bowl for no more than 3 days in a row. For anemia, small dried fish (*iriko*), may be taken, sautéed in a little water or oil with shoyu at the end, 2 small pieces a day.

• **Fruit:** None the best, the less the better, including temperate as well as tropical, until the condition improves. If cravings develop, a small volume of cooked fruit, especially apples, with a pinch of salt or dried fruit may be taken. Avoid all fruit juices and cider.

• **Sweets and Snacks:** Avoid all sweets and desserts, including good quality macrobiotic desserts until the condition improves. Just a little sugar, chocolate, carob, honey, maple syrup, or soy milk will increase viral activity and bring out symptoms. To satisfy a sweet taste, use sweet vegetables every day in cooking, drink sweet vegetable drink (see special drinks below), and sweet vegetable jam. Mochi, rice balls, sushi, and other grain-based snacks may be eaten frequently. Limit rice cakes, popcorn, and other dry or baked snacks as they may cause tightening. In the event of cravings, a small volume of grain-based sweeteners such as barley malt or rice syrup may be taken.

• **Nuts and Seeds:** Nuts and nut butters are to be avoided due to their high amount of fat and protein, except for chestnuts. Unsalted, roasted seeds such as squash seeds and pumpkin seeds may be consumed as a snack, up to 1 cup altogether per week. Sunflower seeds may be taken only in the summer.

• **Seasonings:** Seasonings, such as unrefined sea salt, shoyu, and miso, are to be used moderately to avoid unnecessary thirst. Avoid *mirin* (a sweet cooking wine) and garlic. If you become particularly thirsty after the meal or between meals, you should cut back on these seasonings until normal thirst returns. Do not add shoyu to food at the table.

• **Beverages:** Beverages and other dietary practices can follow the general recommendations, including bancha twig tea as the main beverage. Strictly avoid all aromatic, stimulant beverages, and refrain from grain coffee for the first two to three months.

The most important thing in connection with dietary practice is chewing very well, until all food becomes liquid in the mouth and well mixed with saliva. Chew very very, well, at least 50 times, preferably 100 times per mouthful. It is also important to avoid overeating and eating within 3 hours of sleeping.

Persons who have received or who are currently undergoing medical treatment may need to make further dietary modifications. Please consult your medical doctor, nutritionist, or other healthcare professional.

Special Drinks and Preparations

There are several special drinks and condiments that help strengthen the natural immune function including ume-sho-bancha, ume-sho-kuzu, sweet vegetable drink, lotus root-carrot-kombu-aduki condiment, baked kombu-sesame-shiitake condiment, and umeboshi plums. Please see the chapter on AIDS in *The Cancer Prevention Diet* (revised edition, 1994) by Michio Kushi and Alex Jack for recipes and consult a qualified macrobiotic teacher for guidance.

Home Cares

For a small number of cases, a compress, poultice, or other external application may be needed to help neutralize the infection or gradually help draw out excess mucus and fat from the body.

Miso—fermented soybean paste—is particularly effective in helping to neutralize the spread of viruses and bacteria and prevent infection. In addition to being taken internally in the form of miso soup, it may be used externally as a compress.

"More than four thousand years ago the Chinese routinely treated skin wounds and infectins with a paste made from moldy soybeans," explains Jeffrey A. Fisher, M.D., in his book *The Plague Makers: How We Are Creating Catastrophic New Epidemics—And What We Must Do to Avert Them.* "Almost identical remedies are described in the Hebrew Talmud. . . . The ancient practices all had as a common denominator the use of fermented grains, with molds, yeast and fungi as the fermenting agents.

"Until the 1960s, when scientists at pharmaceutical companies began developing synthetic versions of antibiotics, the naturally produced ones were derived from similar sources: molds, sewage or soil. As the bacteria or fungi producing these early antibiotics have been around for millions of years, it is likely that the pastes, packs or liquids used by these early healers contained antibiotics in some form."

Please read *Basic Home Remedies* by Michio Kushi (One Peaceful World Press, 1994) for the most recent information on the application of these home cares and see a qualified macrobiotic teacher for guidance.

• **Body Scrub:** A body scrub is recommended for everyone. To peform: scrub the whole body once or twice a day including the abdominal region and the spinal region with a towel that has been immersed in hot water and squeezed out. This is helpful for better circulation of blood, lymph, and other body fluids, as well as for activating physical and mental energies.

• **Medical Attention:** If the condition worsens, other lack of improvement is experienced, or a serious, potentially life-threatening condition develops, medical attention is necessary. A medical doctor or other appropriate healthcare professional should be consulted.

Way of Life Suggestions

• Live each day happily without worry
• Walk outdoors every day for a half hour or longer
• Keep green plants in the home to freshen the air
• Wear 100 percent cotton clothing next to the skin, and use cotton sheets and pillowcases
• Avoid or limit watching television, using computers, or exposure to other artificial electromagnetic fields
• A few minutes each day, meditate, pray, or visualize, especially healthy, positive thoughts and images
• Practice safe sex. During intercourse, mucus and other fluids and energies, including the HIV virus, are discharged and exchanged. Natural infection easily arises as a result unless both sides are eating very well
• Strictly avoid all drug use
• Maintain a clean, orderly environment and observe sanitary conditions
• Sing a happy song each day.

9

Regeneration of Modern Society

The modern food and agricultural system is a major vehicle for the creation and spread of new epidemics. Antibiotics are regularly fed to cattle and other livestock. As *Newsweek* reminded its readers in a recent cover story, "With every burger and shake, supermicrobes pour into your gut." Milk in particular is a major source of infection as it is allowed by law to contain a certain concentration of up to 80 different antibiotics that are used to treat dairy cows for udder infections. "With every glassful, people swallow a minute amount of several antibiotics," *Newsweek* continued. Despite regulation, government investigators found traces of 64 antibiotics at levels that raise health concerns and which could produce resistant strains in milk drinkers. In a recent study, scientists at Rutgers University found that antibiotics declared safe by the FDA increased the rate at which resistant bacteria developed by 600 to 2,700 percent. The introduction of genetic engineering will substantially increase the threat. The FDA recently approved as safe rBGH, bovine growth hormone, which increases milk production. But it also increases the risk of udder infection and requires farmers to give their dairy cows even more antibiotics.

Overmedicalization has also resulted in the epidemic spread of disease-resistant bacteria. The indiscriminate use of antibiotics, particularly in a hospital or clinical setting, has led to a wave of medically-caused disease. Multiple-drug-resistant tuberculosis has spread around the world, becoming the leading cause of death, and an estimated one in every three persons—1.7 billion people—is a carrier. Every year in the United States today, an estimated 1.5 million patients acquire infections in the hospital—infections unrelated to their original condition—and of these several hundred thousand die. Though virtually unknown to the public, this epidemic spread of medical-caused infectious disease has resulted in the mandatory creation of nosocomial committees in every hospital in the country to safeguard against infection. (*Nosocomial* means medically-caused disease.) Despite such vigilence, the emergence of antibiotic resistant strains of microbes continues to accelerate. For example, some 40 percent of *staphyloccocus aureus*, the bacteria associated with pneumonia, are resistant to all antibiotics but vancomycin. "We know at some point vancomycin will succumb and the bacteria will grow and proliferate unrestrained," a director of the Veterans Administration told *Newsweek*. "It will be like the 1950 and 1960s, when we had nothing to treat this infection, and the mortality rates were as high as 80 percent." Recently microbiologists have discovered that microbes cannot only develop multiple drug resistance quickly, they can also transfer this ability to other microorganisms. "Bacteria have their own Internet," one researcher quipped. They "swap . . . plasmids the way human beings exchange E-mail."

Meanwhile, genetic engineering poses another danger. A biogenetic tomato approved for consumers contains a gene that gives resistance to the antibiotic kanamycin. The tomato will stay fresher longer, but pass this resistance along to consumers. In 1994, just before the tomato was approved, scientists at Michigan State further warned that inserted genes can recombine with natural plant viruses and produce entirely new viruses at a higher rate than expected. "The implication of the research," the *New York Times* reported, ". . . was that engineering plants to be resistant to viruses might lead to entirely new types of viruses that could cause widespread damage to American harvests."

Clearly, humanity is engaged in war against microbes

that it cannot win. The postwar period of "miracle" drugs and vaccines, and pesticides and chemicals, can now be seen for what it truly represents: a brief respite before the development of more virulent pathogens and the spread of more terrifying diseases. Genetic engineering is the midwife of a brave new world of environmentally-engineered plagues totally unimaginable in the past. From an evolutionary view, these developments may be the last round—for *homo sapiens* and many species. The earth as a whole, as Karl Johnson, M.D., observes in an essay in *Emerging Viruses*, is "a progressively immunocompromised ecosystem."

Transforming the Planet

Our species today faces extinction as a result of the the spread of AIDS, MDR tuberculosis, and emerging viral and bacterial epidemics. Everyone may have a close friend or family member who will suffer from one or another of these new plagues. The era of apocalypse—the external threat of nuclear weapons and the internal threat of heart disease and cancer—is receding. Humanity faces attrition—now quick, now slow—at all levels. States are decomposing in the same way that cells are decomposing. Ideals and family values are collapsing at the same rate as red- and white-blood cells, lymph cells, and DNA are losing their integrity. The pace of decline is accelerated by microwave ovens, electric stoves, computer networks, and other vectors of artificial electromagnetic radiation.

To cope with this grave threat to the continued existence of humanity on this planet, a revolutionary transformation in our view and way of life is urgently required. The principles underlying this transformation include the following points:

• It should be understood that the order of the universe is endless, governing all phenomena, including human life and the appearance and disappearance of health and disease.

• Self-reflection and evaluation should recognize that modern industrial civilization has weakened the natural immunity of human beings to the extent that the future of humanity is imperiled.

• It should be understood that the solution for the new epidemics does not deal only with symptoms or with certain microorganisms alone, but involves a comprehensive approach to reconstructing the total health of people living in modern society and preserving the natural environment of which we are a part.

• It should be understood that the total reconstruction of human health cannot be made by present medical treatment or health-care technology, though, in some cases, they can help slow the epidemic spread of disease and relieve suffering. What is needed is a revolutionary change of view, lifestyle, and dietary habits that respect the universal traditions of humanity and the natural environment. The whole challenge of biological degeneration can only be met by a biological and spiritual transformation of humanity.

• It should be understood that for this biological transformation to take place, all spiritual, religious, philosophical, and scientific communities and orientations must cooperate. East and West, North and South must meet. Ancient traditions and modern technologies must work together to create one healthy, peaceful world.

• It should be understood that the headquarters for this biological and spiritual transformation of humanity is the kitchen in every home and the eating place in every community. In most cases, the leaders of this transformation will be women who take responsibility for preparing the daily food for their family and nourishing their children. Everyone— male and female—is encouraged to learn to cook and should actively participate in some aspect of food cultivation, production, or preparation.

• It should also be understood that this transformation will affect all political, economic, cultural, and social systems. These will inevitably be transformed toward a planetary system which will secure the maximum possible health of humankind, ecological balance, and peace in the world.

• It should be recognized that AIDS, tuberculosis, and the new plagues, disastrous as they are, offers humanity an opportunity to self-reflect and build a new world.

Resources and Authors

The **One Peaceful World Society** is an international information network and macrobiotic friendship society. Membership is $30 year for individuals and $50 for families and benefits include the quarterly *One Peaceful World Newsletter*, a free book from One Peaceful World Press, and discounts on books and study materials. To enroll or for information, please contact: One Peaceful World, Box 10, Becket, MA 01223, (413) 623-2322, Fax (413) 623-8827.

The **Kushi Institute** is an educational center for macrobiotic and holistic studies. For information on programs, please contact: Kushi Institute, Box 7, Becket, MA 01223, (413) 623-5741, Fax (413) 623-8827.

Michio Kushi was born in Japan in 1926 and came to the United States in 1949. Over the last forty years, he has lectured and given seminars on health and diet to medical professionals, government officials, and individuals and families around the world, guiding thousands of people to greater health and happiness. He has inspired the creation of the United Nations Macrobiotic Society, advised governments around the world, and led a seminar on AIDS and diet for several hundred medical doctors and World Health Organization representatives in West Africa. Founder and president of the Kushi Institute and One Peaceful World, Michio Kushi is the author of numerous books and makes his home in Brookline, Massachusetts.

Alex Jack teaches macrobiotic healthcare and philosophy at the Kushi Institute and directs the One Peaceful World Society. He is the co-author with Michio Kushi of *The Cancer Prevention Diet, Diet for a Strong Heart,* and *One Peaceful World.*

Recommended Reading

Ewald, Paul W., *Evolution of Infectious Disease*, Oxford University Press, 1994.

Fisher, Jeffrey A., M.D., *The Plague Makers*, Simon & Schuster, 1994.

Gallo, Robert, M.D., *Virus Hunting: AIDS, Cancer, and the Human Retrovirus*, New Republic/Basic Books, 1991.

Jack, Alex, *Let Food Be Thy Medicine*, One Peaceful World Press, 1994.

Jack, Gale and Alex, *Amber Waves of Grain: American Macrobiotic Cooking*, Japan Publications, 1992.

Kushi, Aveline and Alex Jack, *Aveline Kushi's Complete Guide to Macrobiotic Cooking*, Warner Books, 1985.

Kushi, Michio, *Basic Home Remedies*, One Peaceful World Press, 1994.

Kushi, Michio, *Standard Macrobiotic Diet*, One Peaceful World Press, 1991.

Kushi, Michio, and Martha Cottrell, M.D., with Mark Mead, *AIDS, Macrobiotics, and Natural Immunity* , Japan Publications, 1990.

Kushi, Michio and Edward Esko, *Holistic Health Through Macrobiotics*, Japan Publications, 1993.

Kushi, Michio and Alex Jack, *The Cancer Prevention Diet*, St. Martin's Press, 1993.

Lappé, Marc, *When Antibiotics Fail: Restoring the Ecology of the Body*, North Atlantic Books, 1986.

Monte, Tom, *The Way of Hope: Michio Kushi's Anti-AIDS Program*, New York, Warner Books, 1990.

Morse, Stephen S., editor, *Emerging Viruses*, Oxford University Press, 1993.

Root-Bernstein, Robert, *Rethinking AIDS: The Tragic Cost of Premature Consensus*, The Free Press, 1993.

Checklist of Risk Factors
for AIDS and the New Epidemics

Higher Risk*
(*If excessive)

Dietary

- Meat
- Poultry and Eggs
- Tuna and Other Fatty Fish
- Milk, Butter, Cheese, Yogurt, Ice Cream, and Dairy
- Margarine, Salad Dressing, Spreads, Deep-Fried, and Other Oily, Fatty Foods
- Refined Flour, Yeasted Bread, Baked Products
- Tropical Fruit and Juice, especially Banana, Papaya, Mango, Avocado, Kiwi
- Tomatoes, Potatoes, Pepper, and Tropical Vegetables
- Sugar, Chocolate, Carob, Honey, and Other Sweets
- Soft Drinks; Sparkling, Distilled, Chemicalized Waters
- Spices and Aromatic, Stimulant Herbs
- Coffee, Tea, Tobacco
- Strong Alcohol and Wine
- Canned, Dyed, Frozen, or Sprayed Food
- Food Containing Additives, Preservatives, or Chemicals

Lower Risk

Dietary

- Whole Grains
- Beans
- Tofu, Tempeh, Natto, and Other Soybean Products
- Vegetables
- Sea Vegetables
- Sea Salt, Miso, Shoyu, and Other Natural Seasonings
- Sesame, Corn, and Other Unrefined Oils
- White-Meat Fish
- Temperate-Climate Fruit
- Seeds and Nuts
- Snacks and Desserts Sweetened with Barley Malt, Rice Syrup, or Amasake
- Spring or Well Water
- Nonaromatic, Nonstimulant Teas and Other Traditional Beverages
- Organically Grown Foods
- Naturally Processed Foods
- Locally Grown Foods
- Foods Prepared in Season

Higher Risk*
(*If Excessive)

- Vitamins, Supplements
- Irradiated Food
- Genetically Altered Food

Lifestyle

- Microwave Cooking
- Electrical Cooking
- Non-Stick Cookware
- Bottle-Feeding
- Caesarean Section
- Sedentary Lifestyle
- Prescription Drugs
- Antibiotics
- Anesthetics
- Vaccinations
- Marijuana and Drugs
- Tonsillectomy, Appendectomy, or Other Surgery
- X-Rays, MRI and CAT Scans
- Mercury Amalgam Fillings
- Artificial Radiation from Computers, Television, Cellular Telephones, etc.
- Synthetic Clothing
- Promiscuous Sex

Environmental

- Unclean, Disorderly Home
- Hot, Warm Climate
- High Temperature
- High Humidity
- Spring and Summer
- Urban Environment
- Acid Rain
- Ozone Depletion
- Nuclear and Toxic Waste
- Air Pollution and Excessive CO_2

Lower Risk

Lifestyle

- Gas Cooking
- Wood Cooking
- Stainless Steel and Ceramic Cookware
- Breast-feeding
- Natural Childbirth
- Active Lifestyle
- Daily Walking
- Light to Moderate Exercise
- Farming or Gardening
- Massage or Shiatsu
- Yoga or Martial Arts
- Swimming, Sports, Hobbies
- Meditation, Visualization, Prayer, Self-Reflection
- Singing, Dancing, and Listening to Harmonious Music
- Reading Books and Poems
- Cotton, Natural Fabrics
- Safe Sex

Environmental

- Clean, Orderly Home
- Cold, Cool Climate
- Low Temperature
- Low Humidity
- Fall and Winter
- Rural or Small Town Environment
- Adequate Sunshine
- Green Plants Indoors
- Fresh Air and More Oxygen

From *AIDS and Beyond* by Michio Kushi and Alex Jack
One Peaceful World Press, © 1995.